Essential Oils for Health

100 Amazing and Unexpected Uses for Tea Tree Oil, Peppermint Oil, Eucalyptus Oil, Lavender Oil, and More

Kymberly Keniston-Pond, CIR, CFR, CCMA

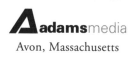
Avon, Massachusetts

Published by
Adams Media, a division of F+W Media, Inc.
57 Littlefield Street, Avon, MA 02322. U.S.A.
www.adamsmedia.com

ISBN 10: 1-4405-8777-9
ISBN 13: 978-1-4405-8777-1
eISBN 10: 1-4405-8778-7
eISBN 13: 978-1-4405-8778-8

Printed in the United States of America.

10   9   8   7   6   5   4   3   2   1

Library of Congress Cataloging-in-Publication Data
Keniston-Pond, Kymberly.
    Essential oils for health / Kymberly Keniston-Pond, CIR, CFR, CCMA.
        pages cm
    ISBN 978-1-4405-8777-1 (pb) -- ISBN 1-4405-8777-9 (pb) -- ISBN 978-1-4405-8778-8 (ebook) --
ISBN 1-4405-8778-7 (ebook)
    1. Essences and essential oils--Therapeutic use. I. Title.
    RM666.A68K46 2015
    615.3'6--dc23
                    2015003283

Many of the designations used by manufacturers and sellers to distinguish their products are claimed as trade-marks. Where those designations appear in this book and F+W Media, Inc. was aware of a trademark claim, the designations have been printed with initial capital letters.

The various uses of essential oils as health aids are based on tradition, scientific theories, or limited research. They often have not been thoroughly tested in humans, and safety and effectiveness have not yet been proven in clinical trials. Some of the conditions for which essential oils can be used as a treatment or remedy are potentially serious, and should be evaluated by a qualified healthcare provider.

This book is intended as general information only, and should not be used to diagnose or treat any health condition. In light of the complex, individual, and specific nature of health problems, this book is not intended to replace professional medical advice. The ideas, procedures, and suggestions in this book are intended to supplement, not replace, the advice of a trained medical professional. Consult your physician before adopting any of the suggestions in this book, as well as about any condition that may require diagnosis or medical attention. The author and publisher disclaim any liability arising directly or indirectly from the use of this book.

Cover design by Michelle Roy Kelly.
Cover image © iStockphoto.com/botamochi.

This book is available at quantity discounts for bulk purchases.
For information, please call 1-800-289-0963.

CONTENTS

Chapter 4: Mental and Spiritual Wellness   **84**

PART 3: BEAUTY   97

Chapter 5: Skincare and Haircare   **98**

Dedication

First I dedicate this book to my handsome, funny, kind, supportive husband, Mark! You really are the "Wind Beneath My Wings" ;-) Love you.

Second, I dedicate this book to you, the reader, for your investment of time. May it prove to be a most serendipitous of beginnings in the beautiful world of aromatherapy.

Acknowledgments

I thank my "Bestie" Debra, and my loving mother Joan for their tireless support, enthusiasm, and encouragement! I appreciate your sacrifice of time to listen, answer, and suggest options for me.

I will always be thankful for being the daughter of my handsome father, Allen, whom I miss every single day. He loved to read and would read only nonfiction. I think he would read this book. Before his death he encouraged me to keep my sense of humor through life, so within these pages I honor his request.

I thank my handsome nephew, Gage, for our fun texts back and forth to get a great blend created!

My beautiful niece, Jazlin, I thank you for using a couple of the blends created and letting me know how they worked.

I thank my two other nieces, Emily and Jovanna, along with their mother, Pattina, for being willing "guinea pigs" using products and giving feedback!

I thank my sister-in-law, Gina, for her visit during the writing of this book and allowing me to blend one of the recipes created to help her sleep!

I thank my husband's children and their spouses, Jonathan and Brittany, Elizabeth and John, and Ben for their support, enthusiasm and understanding of the time I needed to complete this book. Now we can see more of each other!

I also want to thank my editors, Jackie, Peter, and K.J. Fallon, for finding me and presenting to me this awesome opportunity to write about the beautiful gifts of essential oils. I enjoyed this beautiful journey editing with all of you.

I appreciate my fellow colleagues, friends, and family for their excitement and patience as I focused on this book at the expense of not being a willing participant at certain functions. Thank you!

INTRODUCTION

What do Cleopatra, who enticed kings; Queen Esther of Persia, who saved her people from annihilation; and Queen Zenobia of Palmyra have in common? A love affair . . . with essential oils!

These women were not only beautiful from their use of essential oils, but they took the time to learn how to use them to add strength of mind, capture the interest of their husbands and lovers, reduce joint pain, support their bodies through a detox after overindulging in food and drink, and many more remedies.

Today there is a growing interest in essential oils for their therapeutic, emotional, and energetic properties. In fact, you can get an overload of information that at times contradicts itself. How do you use these oils? Do you ingest them or not? Can you use them randomly on the skin without diluting? What if you are under a doctor's supervision and on medication—are there any contraindications? How do you store essential oils? How long will they last? From what part of the plant do you get the oils? How are these parts processed? How do you know you are purchasing pure essential oils? These and many more questions will be addressed in this book in an ethical, unbiased way.

You will find a large number of essential oils to be antibacterial, antifungal, anti-inflammatory, antiseptic, analgesic, carminative, antirheumatic, cell rejuvenating, skin enhancing, and much more. On the emotional and energetic side they stimulate creativity, calm the mind, lessen panic attacks, uplift, cleanse negative thoughts, quiet the mind . . . the list goes on.

In this book you will become intimate with twelve essential oils: clary sage, clove, eucalyptus, frankincense, geranium, ginger, lavender, lemon, peppermint, rosemary, tea tree, and ylang ylang. These are common and affordable. There are more than 100 simple, yet effective recipes to use in your daily life. Learn how one essential oil can support you on many levels.

You don't have to be a queen to have a love affair with essential oils, but you can feel like one as you use them. Turn the page and let your love affair with essential oils begin!

THE MANY HEALTH BENEFITS OF ESSENTIAL OILS

What Is an Essential Oil?

An essential oil is extracted from the flowers, leaves, roots, bark, fruit, resins, seeds, needles, or twigs of a plant or tree. A variety of methods are used to extract the oil, the most widespread form being steam distillation. After the extraction, the liquid on top of the water is the highly concentrated "oil" that will have the aroma of the plant along with all therapeutic properties particular to that plant. The liquid on the bottom is the "hydrosol," which is a diluted but equally important property. The oil on top is 100 percent pure, 100 percent natural, and contains the full therapeutic, emotional, and energetic properties of the plant. Make sure the oil you purchase is not adulterated. Because the oil is highly concentrated, you will need only a few drops to produce the results you intend. In this case, less is more. Essential oils are not "oily" and thus are volatile, meaning they will evaporate, so be sure to recap the bottle when you're done using it.

What Is a Carrier Oil?

A carrier oil is extracted from the portion of the plant that is fat—usually the seed, kernel, or nut. Each carrier oil has its own therapeutic properties, making these an integral and complementary part of a blend. Some common carrier oils are jojoba, grape seed, coconut, rosehip seed, avocado, apricot kernel, and castor. These are "oily" and will not evaporate.

Why Do They Need Each Other?

Just as when making another kind of purchase, you need a "carrier" to transport the goods, since they will "disappear" if unattended. The carrier you use will need to fit the specifics of your purchase. An important reason to use a carrier oil is that essential oils are volatile; they will quickly evaporate. Each carrier oil has its own therapeutic properties that will enhance or support the essential oil once it is delivered. There are a few essential oils that do not need a carrier, and these will be addressed in a later section of the book.

Safely Respect These Beautiful Gifts

By showing due respect for the concentration of chemical properties in pure essential oils, you can positively incorporate them into your daily life. To use them successfully, you must know how to use them safely. Please note the following guidelines:

- Do not use the following oils if you have or are suspected of being vulnerable to epileptic seizures: camphor, fennel, hyssop, rosemary, lavandin, sage, spike lavender, and thuja. These can be too stimulating to the nervous system.
- Essential oils must be stored in dark, airtight glass bottles. When exposed to light, oxygen, and heat, the properties of the oils begin to break down, and they become irritating to the skin. If stored properly, they may last seven to ten years, although this varies. Citrus oils are an exception—they should be kept only one to two years. All oils need to be kept at temperatures between 45°F–65°F. If you notice your citrus oils becoming "cloudy," they are going bad.
- Use oils very cautiously during pregnancy and while breastfeeding. Essential oils can be used during these times but *only* under the guidance of a certified aromatherapist and/or medical professional with accurate knowledge of essential oils. Oils should always be a 1 percent dilution during pregnancy.
- Do not use hyssop oil if you have high blood pressure.
- For children, the elderly, pregnant women, or people with severe health challenges, always use a dilution rate of 1 percent, which is a total of 5–6 drops per 1 ounce (2 tablespoons/30 mL) of carrier oil. A gentler approach is to use hydrosols.
- Always dilute essential oils in a carrier oil before applying to the skin. You may experience a skin tingling or a burning sensation. If this happens,

immediately apply a carrier oil to the affected area and wipe off. Lavender and tea tree are generally safe to use directly on the skin.

- Many citrus oils, including bergamot, as well as cumin, opoponax, angelica root, rue, lemon verbena, and tagetes, cause photosensitivity. Sunlight or sun bed rays must be avoided for at least 12 hours after application unless you wear protective clothing. These oils applied to the skin in *any* dilution may increase the chance of severe burns from the ultraviolet light.
- Do not put essential oils around the eyes or near orifices. If an essential oil does contact these areas, immediately flush with a carrier oil and wipe off the excess. (Plain water will not mix with essential oils. A fatty oil (carrier) can be used, or if you want to use saline solution drops, that will work. A carrier oil will take a bit longer to pull the essential oil out of the eye, but it is safer.)If irritation persists, seek medical attention.
- Persons with allergies to perfumes or who have asthma need to proceed cautiously with oils.
- Application of essential oils to the skin or fur of animals should be done *very* cautiously, especially with cats. Please contact a certified aromatherapist who works with animals for guidance.
- There is a time and place for oral ingestion but *only* with guidance from a certified clinical aromatherapist and medical professional with proper knowledge of essential oils. Essential oils not only can burn the skin without proper dilution, but can also damage the stomach, mouth, and internal organs.
- Keep all essential oils out of the reach of children; they can be poisonous if swallowed.

Specific Essential Oils

We will now look at the oils you will be using in this book. This is a general overview; more details about each essential oil are given throughout the book. Unless otherwise noted:

- Do not use with babies and children under the age of seven.
- If you are pregnant and/or breastfeeding, do not use essential oils without consulting with a certified clinical aromatherapist in this field and/or medical personnel with an essential oils background.

Clary Sage–*Salvia sclarea*

This lovely oil is steam distilled from the flower buds. It is known for supporting a woman both physically and emotionally. Clary sage has a sweet, floral aroma that blends well with geranium and lavender. Therapeutically, clary sage is an antidepressant, antispasmodic (relieves spasms and cramps), antiseptic (assists in fighting germs and infections), and a carminative (a tonic for digestion challenges). This oil can get stagnant energy moving, calm the mind, and stimulate creativity. It assists with indecisiveness and calms nervous anxiety, thus supporting emotional and energetic challenges. Clary sage has the possibility of being a mild irritant to both skin and membranes.

Clove Bud–*Eugenia caryophyllata*

Clove is a warming oil extracted from the flower buds and leaves of the plant using steam distillation. The warmth of clove can reduce pain and strengthen the whole body. This oil is used for colds and flu, along with digestive challenges. Clove blends well with lavender and ginger and is an effective combination should you feel a cold coming. If you feel a bit fatigued, this is a wonderful spicy and warm oil to just inhale for an uplifting effect, but also can be used in a synergy blend. Some therapeutic properties include analgesic (numbs pain), antifungal, antirheumatic (relieves rheumatic pain/swelling), bactericidal (destroys bacteria), and carminative (settles digestion). The warmth and spice of this oil will comfort both body and mind, adding to your self-confidence. ***Do not use*** if you have a blood clotting disorder. ***Do not apply*** on the skin in a bath. ***Keep away from*** children under the age of 2. Use a 1 percent dilution of one drop per 1 teaspoon of carrier oil.

Eucalyptus–*Eucalyptus globulus*

Eucalyptus is a splendid, powerful oil, steam distilled from the plant's leaves and twigs. The aroma is both clean and cleansing. Eucalyptus blends well with lavender and rosemary. Therapeutically eucalyptus is a decongestant, antiviral, antibacterial, and analgesic (numbs pain), and relieves muscle aches and pains. Emotionally and energetically eucalyptus is uplifting, cooling, and cleansing for negative emotions. It helps with concentration and clears the mind. There are many varieties of eucalyptus with different therapeutic, emotional, and energy qualities, so do proper research on the Latin name before you purchase. ***Do not use*** around the face of children under 10. If you have skin challenges, be sure to dilute 1 percent in a carrier oil (1 drop per 1 teaspoon). This is a very potent oil, so 1 drop is 1 drop! Less is more.

Frankincense–*Boswellia carterii*

The frankincense tree is tapped to release the sap, which is then dried as resin. This resin then can be used directly as an incense or distilled to produce the essential oil. Frankincense is a beautiful skin oil for dry, aging skin and helps reduce scar tissue. The aroma is warm, earthy, and sweet. It will blend well with citrus oils, lavender, and rose. Therapeutically, it is analgesic (numbs pain), anti-inflammatory, antiseptic (fights germs and pulmonary infections), carminative, cicatrisant (rejuvenates cells and heals scars), expectorant (removes mucus from respiratory system), and immunostimulant (stimulates immune system). It supports emotional and energetic healing on all levels. Frankincense will quiet your mind, bringing focused attention and tranquility.

Geranium–*Pelargonium graveolens*

This lovely geranium oil is steam distilled from the leaves. A variety of geranium plants are grown around the world, so be sure to research the one you would like to use. The **Geranium-*Pelargonium graveolens*** used in this book, is a "woman's oil" because it can help balance hormones. Geranium blends well with all the oils discussed in this book. Therapeutically, it is an antidepressant, antiseptic, antibacterial, diuretic, anti-inflammatory (cooling), and antispasmodic. Emotionally and energetically, it supports intimate communication, increases intuition and imagination, and opens up the sensory world. The oil can cause skin irritation and should ***not*** be ingested.

Ginger–*Zingiber officinale*

Ginger oil is steam distilled from the plant rhizomes or from fresh ginger. Used for nausea, it is great for stimulating circulation to the areas used. The warming qualities of ginger make it suitable for winter blends. Therapeutically, ginger is analgesic (numbs pain), anti-inflammatory, antiseptic, carminative, diaphoretic (promotes perspiration to support the elimination of waste from the skin), antiemetic (reduces nausea/vomiting), and an expectorant. Its emotional and energetic qualities will support stability, stimulate willpower, and combat burnout. Ginger may irritate the skin; therefore use at a 1 percent dilution when applying to the skin, using in the bath, or in massage oils.

Lavender–*Lavandula angustifolia*

There are a variety of lavenders, so be sure to check out the Latin name and do proper research before purchasing and/or using. The lavender used in this book is **Lavandula angustifolia**. This is one of the most widely known, loved, and adulterated oils worldwide. Be sure to purchase from a highly reputable company to prevent receiving a diluted oil with lots of "chemical" aromas. If there is one oil you want to begin with, lavender is it, due to the variety of applications. Therapeutically, lavender is an antidepressant, antiseptic, hemostatic (stops bleeding), antibacterial, and anti-inflammatory. It is excellent for cleaning wounds, healing burns, and as a sedative. This is just the beginning of its therapeutic value. Emotionally and energetically, it will calm, soothe, nurture, reduce anxiety/fear, alleviate panic attacks, and bring balance to all body systems. It is a safe oil to use, being nontoxic and a nonirritant.

Lemon–*Citrus limon*

This oil is pressed from the outer rind of the fruit. The aroma is amazingly fresh and clean. It blends well with all citrus oils, eucalyptus, frankincense, lavender, rosemary, and ylang ylang. Therapeutically, it is an antiseptic (fights germs/infections/flu/colds/bronchitis), a bactericide, disinfectant (for cleaning), and is used for oily skin and for boils. Emotionally and energetically, think of the "happy face" . . . bright yellow! This oil is full of outward, expanding energy. You will simultaneously feel uplifted and cleansed. This oil is photosensitive, meaning it can react to the sunlight and cause burning and skin damage. If you use this oil in skincare preparation, be sure to cover up when going outside. Also, citrus oils easily oxidize (or become rancid) and thus will cause skin irritation.

Peppermint–*Mentha x piperita*

Peppermint is steam distilled from leaves. The aroma is minty and warm yet stimulating. Peppermint blends well with eucalyptus, lavender, lemon, and rosemary. Peppermint and lavender beautifully complement each other. Therapeutically, peppermint is analgesic, anti-inflammatory, antiseptic, antispasmodic, carminative, cooling (helps reduce itching), a febrifuge (reduces fever), decongestant, expectorant, and a liver protector. Emotionally and energetically, it is uplifting, awakening, and clears energy. Peppermint stimulates creativity and new ideas and also supports self-confidence. This oil may be a skin irritant; do not keep close to other homeopathic remedies, as it may null the effectiveness of them. Use in a dilution of 1 percent. ***Do not*** apply on or near the face of babies and children under five. The oil is more therapeutic in small doses.

Rosemary–*Rosmarinus officinalis*

Rosemary is steam distilled from the flowering tips and leaves of the plant. Rosemary is used in our culinary endeavors for flavoring and as an antioxidant. The aroma is fresh and sharp, and immediately puts a smile on your face. It blends nicely with lavender, peppermint, and all citrus oils. Therapeutically, it is an astringent (tightens and tones the skin), anti-bacterial (for acne, dermatitis, eczema, and athlete's foot); antispasmodic, diuretic, analgesic; a stimulant for the nervous system when loss of smell occurs; carminative; and a stimulant for memory. Emotionally and energetically, it is energizing and uplifting. This oil will stimulate and strengthen the mind, clearing negative thoughts and encouraging clarity. ***Do not use*** if you are pregnant and/or breastfeeding, have epilepsy, other seizure disorders, or fever.

Tea Tree–*Malaleuca alternifolia*

When I think of what to put in my first aid kit, tea tree oil is at the top of the list. It has been used for abscesses, acne, fevers, warts, colds, flu, and for stimulating the immune system. The aroma is medicinal or slightly musty. Tea tree blends well with clary sage, clove, ginger, lemon, and rosemary. Tea tree blended with eucalyptus and geranium is a good combination for fungal infections.

Therapeutically, it is antiseptic, anti-infectious, antifungal, an expectorant, and decongestant. Emotionally and energetically, this oil builds strength, self-confidence, and uplifts the spirit. It may be a skin irritant on sensitive skin. Many people use it "neat" (undiluted); however, if your skin is sensitive then dilute the oil in a small amount of a carrier oil of your choice.

Ylang Ylang–*Cananga odorata*

Ylang ylang is steam distilled from the flowers. It has a beautiful, deeply sweet, sensual aroma. If not blended with a sharp citrus oil like lemon or orange, it can be very overpowering, even nauseating. Therapeutically, ylang ylang is an antidepressant, analgesic, anti-inflammatory, sedative, and nervine (for emotional shock/extreme anxiety or tension). Emotionally and energetically, it will encourage feelings of joy and pleasure, promoting a sensual awareness and relaxation. It is nontoxic and nonirritating; however, please be careful with it if you have low blood pressure.

PART 1

HEALTH

Chapter 1
PHYSICAL WELLNESS

Our physical condition affects every aspect of our lives, and we need to keep a close eye on it. We need to maintain healthy nutrition combined with exercise for endurance, muscle strength, cardiovascular health, and flexibility. Thus, you need to become in tune with and listen to your body and take personal responsibility for your fitness regimen. This will empower you to make wise decisions when eating and in finding the perfect exercise. This in turn will support your self-esteem, self-control, and sense of direction in life. When we physically feel good, we look good. When we look good, we are emotionally energized and mentally alert, which feeds into our spiritual side. Everything works together harmoniously if we make responsible decisions. Ask yourself the following questions about your physical wellness:

- Do I know my important numbers, i.e., cholesterol, weight, blood pressure?
- How is my sleeping pattern?
- Do I get an annual checkup?
- Am I abusing tobacco, alcohol, and/or drugs?
- How many times a week am I exercising?
- How much water am I drinking daily?
- Am I a "binge" eater or do I have regular, small meals throughout the day?

These are just a few questions to help you think about your current state of physical wellness. The following chapters will discuss how essential oils can help with a variety of minor health challenges. The information that follows is not a replacement for professional medical attention.

1. HEARTBURN

It all starts with just one bite. Gastric reflux or indigestion, often referred to as heartburn, is due to stomach acid or sometimes even food from the stomach flowing back into the esophagus. The result is a deep burning sensation or extreme discomfort after eating. Sometimes you may have difficulty swallowing or feel as if food is stuck very low in your esophagus. Some things you can do to manage heartburn include:

■ Stop smoking.
■ Eliminate or limit alcohol intake to one drink per day.
■ Pay attention to what foods may be contributing to heartburn.
■ Slightly elevate your pillow when you sleep.
■ Stop eating two to three hours before bed.
■ Wear loose-fitting clothes.
■ If you are carrying extra weight, work on losing it through exercise and correct nutrition.

Slowly sipping on peppermint tea with a bit of honey may ease the pain. The essential oils of **clove, lavender, peppermint,** and **eucalyptus** can also bring relief. Massaging these oils on the skin (not drinking them) helps to relieve pain, relax the nervous system, and in turn, relax the esophagus. They are anti-inflammatory, as well. While you are preparing your tea, make the following:

HEARTBURN RELIEF

1 teaspoon grape seed oil
1 drop clove (analgesic—numbs pain; carminative—settles digestion. Do not use clove if you have a blood clotting disorder.)
2 drops eucalyptus (analgesic—numbs pain; relieves muscle aches and pains)
2 drops lavender (anti-inflammatory, sedative, relaxing)

Combine all essential oils and blend together. Add combined essential oils to a carrier oil and shake to blend. Massage over upper abdomen in a circular motion.

Make sure to rest in an upward sitting position. Sip slowly on the tea after massaging on the oil blend. Your tea should be warm, not hot.

ESSENTIAL OILS TIP

If you experience heartburn on a daily basis, do not ignore these signals from your body. Sometimes constipation causes feelings of nausea and indigestion. Let your doctor know what is happening and how often.

2. BLOATING

Three top reasons for bloating are overeating, excess gas, and bloat-inducing foods.

▓ Overeating. Eat smaller portions and eat slowly. Chew with intention. Honor your body by giving it the time to send proper satiety signals to the brain. Rich and fatty foods take longer to digest than protein or carbohydrates. Limiting the amount of fats in your daily diet will reduce bloating.

▓ Excess gas is created when you drink through a straw, chew gum, gulp down carbonated drinks, suck on hard candy, or are excessively nervous. Use balance and practice breathing exercises when nervous to reduce taking in more air.

▓ Bloat-inducing food. Beans, lentils, fruits, and certain vegetables (Brussels sprouts, cabbage, cauliflower, carrots, prunes, and apricots) contain sugars and starches that cause excess gas and bloating while they are broken down by the body. When you add whole grain and fiber to your diet, increase your water for the fiber to be absorbed and move at a nice speed through the digestive system.

Let's use the essential oils of **peppermint** and **ginger** to also help combat bloating.

BLOATING BE GONE

2 tablespoons unscented body lotion
3 drops peppermint (analgesic—pain numbing; anti-inflammatory, calms the stomach muscles, eases cramps and stomach aches.)
4 drops ginger (anti-inflammatory, carminative—settles digestion; antiemetic—reduces nausea) Note: Inhaling ginger essential oil is also good for motion sickness.

Thoroughly blend lotion and oils. Massage some of the lotion onto the area of discomfort and some onto the bottom of each foot all across the arch and down.

ESSENTIAL OILS TIP

If you anticipate bloating while away from home, add 2 drops peppermint essential oil and 2 drops clove essential oil onto a cotton ball. Place the ball into a zip lock plastic bag and carry it with you. If the need arises, open the bag and inhale from the ball. This will provide some immediate relief.

3. CONSTIPATION

Excreting is important since it eliminates toxic waste from our body. If you experience fewer than three bowel movements per week, you are constipated. If you experience less than one per week, you have acute constipation. If you are seeing blood, experiencing abdominal pain, cramps, nausea, vomiting, or involuntary loss of weight, immediately see your doctor.

Among the reasons for constipation are hormonal imbalance, medications, overuse of stimulating laxatives, poor diet, poor bowel habits, disruption of daily routine, lack of activity, stress, and not drinking enough water.

You can make some changes to get the body back in "motion":

▦ Add 2 tablespoons of ground flaxseed to your daily diet.
▦ Add one prune a day to your diet. They come packaged separately and conveniently now!
▦ Drink 2–4 glasses of *warm* water each day.
▦ Walk 30 minutes a day.

Rosemary, lemon, and **peppermint** oils can bring relief, stimulate the colon, and help get things moving!

LET'S MOVE IT

2 tablespoons grape seed oil

4 drops rosemary (antispasmodic, carminative) (Do not use rosemary if you are pregnant and/or breastfeeding, prone to seizures,or have epilepsy.)

3 drops lemon (carminative, expels gas from intestines)

3 drops peppermint (analgesic, antispasmodic, carminative)

Thoroughly blend all oils and massage over the lower back and lower abdomen. You can also add 3 drops of this blend to a castor oil pack.

ESSENTIAL OILS TIP

Here is an easy way to do a castor oil pack. Apply approximately ¼ cup of organic castor oil over your lower abdomen. Lay a thin cloth over the top of the oil. Then, add plastic on top of the cloth to create a barrier. Finally, place a hot water bottle or heating pad on top of the plastic and rest for approximately 45 minutes. After resting, remove all of the plastic and cloth. You can wash off the excess oil, or just leave it on to nourish your colon. Use a castor oil pack for 2 days in a row then hold off for 2 days. Repeat for up to 2 weeks and when you feel your body balancing, then you can just do a maintenance pack once a week.

4. FLATULENCE

Gas builds up in your digestive system. Your body needs to expel this gas and sooner or later it comes out in a fart or a fluff. Everyone does it every day depending on our lifestyle of diet and exercise. What causes this? We take in too much air by chewing gum, smoking, gulping our food and beverages, and as a result of some foods and medications. If you are taking such a medication, do not stop taking it but talk with your doctor about things that can help you with the resulting gas.

We'll use a combination of **ginger, lavender,** and **peppermint** to address flatulence.

THE FLUFFERNATOR

1 teaspoon grape seed oil
2 drops ginger (anti-inflammatory, carminative—settles digestion)
3 drops lavender (anti-inflammatory, analgesic—numbs pain; calming)
1 drop peppermint (analgesic, antispasmodic, carminative)

Thoroughly blend oils. Massage over abdomen including the navel and lower colon area.

5. HIATAL HERNIA

The diaphragm lies between the abdomen and chest with the stomach being below the diaphragm. In some people, a part of their stomach will push through the diaphragm by means of the hiatus into the chest resulting in a hiatal hernia.

The most common symptoms of a hiatal hernia are heartburn, which increases when bending over; pain when swallowing; some chest pain; and lots of burping. If, however, you experience nausea, vomiting and/or your body will not allow you to relieve the gas or have a bowel movement, seek medical attention immediately.

Acid reflux and heartburn usually are treated with over-the-counter antacids or receptor blockers to lower the amount of acid. You can reduce the symptoms by eliminating spicy foods, tomatoes, caffeine, alcohol, and citrus fruits. It would also be helpful to stop smoking, sleep with the head slightly elevated, and after you eat, don't bend over. It may be helpful to lose excess weight, ask for help with lifting heavy items, and if you find you are straining with bowel movements, drink more water.

To address this with essential oils, we'll use **ginger, lavender,** and **rosemary**.

HIATAL HERNIA HELP

2 tablespoons grape seed oil

6 drops ginger (numbs pain, anti-inflammatory, settles digestive challenges, reduces nausea/vomiting)

6 drops lavender (anti-inflammatory, sedative, relaxing)

5 drops rosemary (antispasmodic, pain reducing, settles digestive challenges)

Do not use rosemary if you are pregnant and/or nursing, are prone to seizures, or have epilepsy.

Thoroughly blend oils. Massage over esophagus, chest, and upper stomach area. Reapply as needed.

ESSENTIAL OILS TIP

While you are preparing your recipe, take a moment and inhale the fragrance of each oil separately before adding the drops. Do so with your eyes closed and see how you feel. Pay close attention to the discomfort you are experiencing to discover which oil brings the most relief. Let your body make the choice for you.

6. INTESTINAL SPASMS/CRAMPS

You can experience intestinal spasms and cramps as a result of excessive gas in the intestines. This is due, in a large part, to food. Bad combinations of foods can create agony. Stress can also affect us when we eat.

First things first: Remove *all* tight clothing immediately. Drink lots of warm water to get things "moving." Breathe deeply to calm down. Massage your lower intestines to help get things going and deal with the uncomfortable pain. We will keep the oil recipe very simple since the pain will not allow you to do too much thinking.

Clove, ginger, and **peppermint** will help soothe the digestive tract and bring relief.

INTESTINAL RELIEF

1 tablespoon castor oil

1 tablespoon grape seed oil

4 drops clove (analgesic—numbs pain; carminative—settles digestion)

6 drops ginger (calms the digestive system; an antiseptic, laxative, and stimulant)

4 drops peppermint (relaxes the digestive tract, relieves diarrhea and/or constipation, calms cramps and spasms)

Thoroughly bend all the oils. Massage over the lower abdomen and directly over the areas of pain and spasms. Be sure to walk around as this will help the body expel the excess gas.

ESSENTIAL OILS TIP

Omit the clove if you have a blood clotting disorder.

7. ALLERGIES . . . HAY FEVER

The term "hay fever" can be a bit misleading since there is usually no hay causing the allergy and no fever along with it. Because it generally happens in spring and summer a more correct term might be "seasonal allergic rhinitis" or SAL. Between the growth of grasses, trees, weeds, and other plants, and windy weather, pollen counts vary from day to day. The higher the pollen count, the more likely the allergen will affect you. Other allergens caused by pets, mold, and fungi fall under this heading. Everyone is affected differently, but there are common symptoms of which to be aware:

- Lots of sneezing
- Very itchy nose, ears, and eyes, which may be bloodshot
- Runny nose
- Nasal and sinus congestion
- Pressure inside the head, making concentration difficult

Allergy medicines, including antihistamines, help control the histamine being released from your immune system. However, these medications can cause drowsiness. We can turn to essential oils to bring some relief. Eucalyptus is a decongestant, antibacterial, and analgesic. You can do a simple **steam inhalation** by adding **1 drop of eucalyptus** in a bowl of hot water. Drape a large towel over your head while leaning above the steam. Breathe in the eucalyptus steam for a few minutes, keeping your eyes closed. This will begin to open up the respiratory passages quickly.

You can also make a face cream with the following oils:

2 tablespoons unscented face cream
3 drops lavender (natural antihistamine, anti-inflammatory and relaxing)
1 drop peppermint (decongestant, anti-inflammatory)

Thoroughly blend all oils and cream. Use in the morning and evening to provide protection against allergies and nourish your skin. Keep cream away from your eyes.

8. ALLERGIES . . . SKIN RASH

"I can't stop scratching my skin!" Have you ever said this? Maybe you are challenged with dermatitis such as psoriasis, acne, rosacea, or eczema. Any of these skin conditions will cause itching, redness, and pain.

Our skin is the largest organ in the body's system. It's a barrier against the outer world, and as such it takes quite a beating. There are a number of reasons why our skin will react unkindly, including detoxing, which can cause the liver to overload with toxins that the body will expel through the skin. If you are afflicted with a skin rash or irritation, the place to begin is at its origin. How can essential oils give immediate relief?

Let's see how just three will help: **lavender, geranium,** and **tea tree oil**.

ITCH AWAY

1 teaspoon borage oil (soothes irritated and inflamed skin)

5 teaspoons grape seed oil

8 drops lavender (antiseptic, healing, soothing, cooling)

4 drops geranium (promotes blood circulation to the "hot" areas on the skin; improves elasticity

4 drops tea tree (antibiotic, antiseptic, anti-infectious)

Thoroughly blend all oils. Apply directly to the affected area on clean skin.

ESSENTIAL OILS TIP

Lavender is such a soothing essential oil for skin. It can be applied topically "neat" (undiluted) to skin. Please make sure that you are using a *pure* lavender from a reputable company.

9. ALLERGIES . . . SINUS

Springtime comes with two faces—one fresh and beautiful, pregnant earth giving birth to new life; the other producing allergens in the air and battling our hard-working immune systems.

Allergies stem from our over-sensitive immune system trying to protect the body from disease and infections. They will attack substances to which you're allergic (called allergens) the same way as they would a virus or bacteria. When exposed to an allergen the body produces an abundance of histamine causing the cells in the nose and throat to swell and drain fluid down your throat.

Through the allergy season, many people live on antihistamines and decongestants or prescription medication. Others receive allergy shots several times during the year for relief. However, many more people are now looking for a more natural alternative. Two essential oils that may help: **lavender** and **peppermint**. There are several different ways to use them.

Lavender is a natural antihistamine and anti-inflammatory.

1. Add one drop to your cheeks, forehead, and sinuses as needed.

Also, apply 2–3 drops to the bottom of your feet before bed.
2. Apply 1–2 drops into the palms of your hands. Rub your hands together and cup over your nose and deeply inhale 4–6 breaths. You can also place 2–3 drops on a cotton ball, secure in a zip lock bag, and take with you. Inhale 4–5 breaths as needed.

Peppermint has analgesic (pain relief) and anti-inflammatory properties and has been used for centuries to relieve nasal congestion.

1. Apply 1 drop to the back of neck twice a day.
2. Dilute in a carrier oil and apply around your nostrils. Note: Do not apply peppermint oil neat (undiluted) around the nostrils as it will sting the sensitive nasal tissues.
3. Apply 1–2 drops on the palms of your hands. Rub your hands together and cup over your nose and deeply inhale 4–6 breaths. You can also place 2–3 drops on a cotton ball, secure in a zip lock bag, and take with you. Inhale 4–5 times as needed.

10. IRRITABLE BOWEL SYNDROME

Unfortunately, there is no cure for Irritable Bowel Syndrome (IBS). Diet and stress management do, however, seem to moderate it.

Let's talk diet. Try to minimize fried/fatty, spicy, "fluff" (flatulence) inducing foods, and caffeine. Add more fiber to your diet by means of supplements, beans, oatmeal, and some fruits. Gradually introduce the fiber if your body is not used to digesting it. Drink lots of water. Eat smaller portions or do as a cow does and just "graze" throughout the day. Also, if you are a smoker, give serious thought to quitting.

Now, let's mess with stress. Keep a journal and note when your IBS flares up. Pay close attention to what is going on in your life at that time. Were you facing financial, physical, emotional, or career challenges? Eliminate the stresses that can be removed and "breathe" through the ones you cannot change. Focus completely on your breathing. Thoughtful, intentional breathing is holistically calming. Taking a short walk will do wonders.

Some have found relief by drinking peppermint and/or ginger tea, brewed from real peppermint and ginger. These teas have a calming effect on the intestines and relieve gas. **Peppermint** essential oil may prove very effective due to its anti-spasmodic (muscle calming) and analgesic properties. Peppermint is also very settling to the mind. Add 2–3 drops to 1 tablespoon of grape seed oil and massage on the abdomen.

ESSENTIAL OILS TIP

There are no clearly understood causes for IBS and therefore a professional assessment is encouraged.

11. LEG AND FOOT CRAMP RELIEF

Have you ever been walking or sleeping when out of nowhere you are in excruciating pain from your toes, calf, or leg? It can be "breathtaking" and "crippling" all at once, sometimes even bringing tears to your eyes. All you want is instant relief! Thus is the experience of muscle cramps or a charley horse (muscle cramp, usually in the back of the calf).

Some possible causes are:

- Poor circulation
- Dehydration
- Muscle fatigue
- Low levels of magnesium and/or potassium
- Side effects of some medications
- Not stretching adequately before or after exercise

So what can we do that may lower the risks?

- Eat more foods high in magnesium/potassium/calcium
- Increase your water intake
- Properly stretch before and after exercising
- Do not overexert your muscles
- Add a daily walk of 15–30 minutes

For immediate help, you can try massaging, cooling the muscle with ice, or warming the muscle with heat. Also beneficial is to work the muscle by pulling your toes toward your head.

Using the essential oils of **clary sage, lavender, peppermint,** and **rosemary** can make a blend for wonderful, immediate relief.

CRAMP AWAY

2 tablespoons grape seed oil

3 drops clary sage (antispasmodic)

6 drops lavender (anti-inflammatory, analgesic—numbs pain, soothing)

3 drops peppermint (analgesic, antispasmodic, cooling)

3 drops rosemary (analgesic, antispasmodic)

Thoroughly blend all oils. Use directly over area(s) of spasm for relief.

ESSENTIAL OILS TIP

Do not use rosemary if you are pregnant and/or breastfeeding, have epilepsy, or are prone to seizures. Omit rosemary oil from this recipe and increase the drops of lavender by 2.

12. SHINGLES SYNERGY BLEND

Herpes zoster, better known as shingles, is a viral infection of the nerve roots. This does not "play nice" with us when we are children, when it shows up as chickenpox. You may think that it has left your body when all is over and you're feeling better, but it doesn't go away. Herpes zoster can lie dormant inside your body for years before emerging as shingles.

Shingles' symptoms are very different from chickenpox. Before the virus produces any visible signs, you may have headaches, feel as if you have the flu without a fever, and experience sensitivity to light. What you next see and feel on your body is a very painful rash. The essential oils of **eucalyptus, lavender, lemon,** and **tea tree** can be blended for relief.

SHINGLES RELIEF

2 tablespoons fractionated coconut oil—the fatty acid has been separated out, leaving a liquid that will not go rancid, will not stain, and is not greasy (or you can use grape seed)

4 drops eucalyptus (analgesic—numbs pain; antibacterial, antiviral)

4 drops lavender (antiseptic, anti-inflammatory, antibacterial)

4 drops lemon (antiseptic, heals skin)

4 drops tea tree (antifungal, anti-infectious, antiseptic)

Thoroughly blend all oils together.

Use a cotton ball to apply directly to the affected area every 2–3 hours. Continue until blisters/bumps are gone and pain has decreased. If topical application is too painful you can make a body spray in a 4-ounce plastic (PET) bottle. First add 1 teaspoon of Shingle Relief Blend and 1 teaspoon of vegetable glycerin to the bottle. Then add 3½ ounces of distilled water into the bottle. Shake well and lightly spray over affected area. Be sure to add the oils to the bottle before the water.

ESSENTIAL OILS TIP

Lemon is a citrus oil and will oxidize within 1–2 years if not properly stored (in a dark glass bottle, tightly capped and refrigerated). This oil will be cloudy in appearance if it has oxidized and it will not be skin friendly. Therefore, please make sure you are using a *pure* lemon oil that is still fresh.

13. NERVE PAIN

Everything our body does from breathing to feeling to moving is tied into our nervous system. When our body suffers an injury, we immediately feel pain. We need to take very good care of our nerves.

The pain associated with a malfunctioning nervous system is very different from regular pain. You may feel a tingling, burning, or numbness. If the nerve has been damaged, it may take a long time to repair itself; in some cases it will not. One thing is for sure, if you have nerve pain, you know it!

Along with the medical and pain management treatments available, many people have found relief from aromatherapy. The oils of **frankincense, lavender,** and **peppermint** can be blended and used two ways:

- Massage directly over the area of intense pain.
- Use in a warm bath. *After* filling tub with warm water add 6 drops of the synergy blend and relax for 15–20 minutes.

ESSENTIAL OILS TIP

Helichrysum–*Helichrysum italicum* is a beautiful oil that receives much attention for its anti-inflammatory and cell rejuvenating properties. If you search for this oil in its pure form it will be (as of this writing) approximately $65–$75 for 5 mL. Remember, if you take care of your oils (dark bottles tightly closed and refrigerated) they will last for years, and you only use *drops* at a time. This oil is well worth the investment. If you choose to use it for nerve pain you can add 3 drops to the Nerve Pain Relief blend.

14. MUSCLE PAIN

We work, we play, we clean the house, we make time to exercise or try a new form of exercise and our muscles get our attention and say, "Hello!" Then, sometimes we are living with a chronic autoimmune or inflammatory condition similar to osteoarthritis. However our muscles get our attention, there are ways to give them the support that they need.

If your muscles are sore due to overexertion or you're trying a new form of exercise and you really like it, just remember the more you use your muscles, the stronger they become. If you're doing something new, work into it gradually.

If your muscles are sore due to chronic physical challenges, they still need to be moved, but more gently. You will actually notice a difference and feel better upon moving, walking, or stretching.

A note of caution: Should your muscle pain be quick, intense, and last longer than 3 to 4 days or continue to intensify, you may have an injury that needs medical assistance. So, call your doctor when the pain will not go away.

With the topical application of **eucalyptus, ginger,** and **peppermint,** you may find the pain subside.

MUSCLE MASSAGE

2 tablespoons grape seed oil

6 drops eucalyptus (analgesic, pain-numbing)

5 drops ginger (analgesic, anti-inflammatory)

5 drops peppermint (analgesic, anti-inflammatory, anti-spasmodic)

Blend all oils thoroughly. Massage at the point of pain in a circular motion as needed.

You can also add 4 drops of the blend to a hot bath and soak as long as possible. Note: Always add the essential oil blend after you have filled the tub and turned off the water.

ESSENTIAL OILS TIP

You may want to ice the inflamed muscle by wrapping an ice pack (or frozen peas) in a thin towel and placing on the sore spot. A little later you can switch to heat to increase the blood flow to the area. Alternate 15 minutes with ice, 15 minutes with heat.

15. JOINT PAIN

More women than men suffer from joint pain. Causes of joint pain for women vary greatly, including hormones, autoimmune diseases, osteoarthritis, and/or rheumatoid arthritis. This makes it more challenging for women to find relief. A woman's response to pain also differs from a man's; a woman's digestive system works slower as well, thus making any pain medication act at a slower pace.

The pain and discomfort associated with joints can be swelling, redness, warmth (on the joint), and morning stiffness until you get the joint moving. Other pain can come from moving the joint too much.

Seek medical attention if your joint pain is followed or concurrent with a fever, if you experience involuntary weight loss during a period of joint pain, and/or your pain becomes severe and lasts more than two to three days.

Add the following to your daily diet and/or routine:

- Begin walking 10–15 minutes a day and increase when you feel you can.
- Add more magnesium to your diet with leafy greens like spinach and kale along with nuts.
- Turmeric and ginger teas have wonderful anti-inflammatory

properties. Make sure to purchase real turmeric and ginger teas.

The following essential oil blend of **eucalyptus, geranium, frankincense,** and **rosemary** can be applied either directly with massage or as a hot compress.

JOINT PAIN BLEND

2 tablespoons grape seed oil

3 drops eucalyptus (analgesic—numbs pain)

3 drops frankincense (analgesic, anti-inflammatory)

6 drops geranium (anti-inflammatory)

6 drops rosemary (analgesic, antispasmodic)

Thoroughly blend all oils and massage directly on the joint. To make a hot compress: In ¾ cup of hot water add 8 drops of Joint Pain Blend and mix well. Then add a small cloth to absorb all the mixture. Wrap this with some plastic and then a dry cloth. You now have a compress to lay on the painful joint. Leave on for up to 1 hour.

ESSENTIAL OILS TIP

Do not use rosemary oil if you are pregnant and/or breastfeeding, have epilepsy, or are prone to seizures. Omit rosemary oil from this recipe and replace with 6 drops of lavender for the same therapeutic properties.

16. CALCIFIED SPINAL PAIN

As we age, the spinal canal begins to narrow, placing pressure on the spinal cord. This may cause the ligaments in our spine to thicken and harden, a condition known as "calcification." Bones may get larger and we end up with bone spurs or "osteophytes." Some people are born with this, but more commonly as you use your spine throughout life it wears out a little bit. Symptoms vary from individual to individual and may include constant pain, weakness, numbness or cramping in one or both arms/legs, or a shot of pain going down the leg beginning at buttocks (sciatica).

There are medications available for the pain and also surgery for those who choose these routes. A variety of holistic options are now available including chiropractic care, acupuncture, reflexology, and acupressure. You can also gain relief by losing excess weight, becoming a nonsmoker, doing gentle stretching, and paying close attention to your posture.

The essential oils of **peppermint, geranium, ginger, lavender,** and **rosemary** may offer relief in the following recipe:

SPINAL STENOSIS RELIEF

2 tablespoons grape seed oil

3 drops geranium (analgesic—pain numbing; anti-inflammatory, antispasmodic)

3 drops ginger (analgesic, antispasmodic, warming)

4 drops lavender (antispasmodic, anti-inflammatory)

3 drops peppermint (anesthetic, analgesic, anti-inflammatory, cooling)

4 drops rosemary (analgesic, antispasmodic, anti-inflammatory)

Blend all oils together. Massage directly on the area of pain and discomfort. You can also make a hot compress as follows: In ¾ cup of hot water add 8 drops of Spinal Stenosis Relief Blend and mix well. Then, add a small cloth to absorb all the mixture. Wrap this with some plastic and then a dry cloth. You now have a compress to lay on the painful area. Leave on for up to 1 hour.

Note: If the area feels warm, make a *cold compress* by substituting cold water for the hot water.

ESSENTIAL OILS TIP

Do not use rosemary oil if you are pregnant and/or breastfeeding, have epilepsy, or are prone to seizures. Omit rosemary and increase lavender oil by 2 drops.

17. SPINAL STIFFNESS

You wake up, push your covers off and, whoa! . . . your back is so stiff. Upon finally standing up, you think, what can I do? Well, many people begin their day with some slow stretching to warm up the body and spine. Then, they take a nice warm shower and just let the water play upon their stiff body bringing it back to life.

While in the shower, add 2 drops of **eucalyptus** to your shower floor. This will assist with numbing any pain in your muscles and spine. Breathe deeply through the nose to let your brain take the therapeutic properties directly to your spine (and any other place needed). Just relax your body and clear your mind for the day.

After your shower, you can add the following oils to 2 tablespoons of your unscented body lotion:

- 1 drop eucalyptus (analgesic—pain numbing)
- 2 drops geranium (analgesic, anti-spasmodic, anti-inflammatory)
- 1 drop peppermint (analgesic, anesthetic, antispasmodic, anti-inflammatory)

Blend the oils with the cream and massage onto the bottoms of your feet. Pay particular attention to massaging from the big toe all the way down to your heel on the inside of your foot. This is where your spinal reflexes, nerve points, and acupressure points are.

18. TOO LITTLE APPETITE

There are times in your life when you just don't want to eat. This can be due to numerous reasons. Illness, medication, poor diet, or depression can add to your loss of appetite. If you haven't really felt like eating in a while, you should speak with a medical professional to ensure there are no serious underlying causes for concern.

When our bodies become dehydrated, we can lose our appetite. So, begin by drinking more water. Choose nutrient-rich foods, and have smaller meals. Take some time to discover what *you* like to eat and try new flavors. This is a wonderful way to honor yourself!

Aromatherapy can assist you on this journey, both stimulating an appetite and bringing comfort to the soul. Make an **inhaler** to keep with you as you prepare your meals and eat them.

Place the drops of oil directly onto the "wick" of the inhaler. After the oils are absorbed put the wick inside the cap, place the end of the inhaler on the bottom (you will hear it snap closed), then attach the covering over the finished inhaler.

Use your inhaler before meals and while preparing your meals. Unscrew the top of inhaler, press 1 nostril closed with 1 finger, inhale through the other nostril. Then, do the same with the other side. Repeat 1–2 more times. Breathe in through the nostrils and out through the mouth.

ESSENTIAL OILS TIP

Inhalers are a wonderful way to carry your blends with you. You can find these at most essential oil stores in your area.

YUMMIE

5 drops lemon (uplifting and energizing)

3 drops peppermint (clears stagnant energy, stimulates creativity, supports self-confidence)

3 drops ylang ylang (promotes a sensual awareness; very relaxing)

19. TOO MUCH APPETITE

Whatever your personal dietary goals are, using essential oils will complement and support each stage.

How? Through the use of smell. When we inhale anything, it streams immediately to the limbic system. This, in turn, will make you feel good or bad, bringing back memories wanted or unwanted. That's why many realtors have an apple pie baking in an oven during an open house . . . you smell the aroma, feel warm and cozy, and will look at the property with an attitude conducive to making it your home.

Let's examine a few oils and how they will help. The first is **grapefruit,** to stimulate the hypothalamus part of the brain; using this oil will diminish any false urge to eat while helping you feel confident and positive. Keep this close at hand for when cravings try to take control and inhale deeply 3–4 times per nostril. The more you do this, the better it will work.

A lack of self-confidence and self-worth sometimes weighs on us. These negative energies can sabotage any self improvement. **Lemon** comes to the rescue, making you feel cleansed and expanding a positive energy. This is a good oil to always keep on hand for inhaling when you begin to feel negative about yourself. Just follow the inhalation directions for grapefruit.

A healthy eating program will help rid your body of toxins. When you shower, take a couple gulps of the warm water. Your liver eliminates toxins through the skin. Warm water helps the liver push toxins through your skin while showering them down the drain. Here's a simple recipe using only two oils: **rosemary** and **lavender**.

TOXI-GONE

8 tablespoons grape seed oil

15 drops lavender (supports elimination of excess fat)

15 drops rosemary (stimulates liver to support flow of bile; supports metabolism)

Thoroughly blend all oils. After bath or shower, massage over the body using a circular motion. Can be used up to twice per day.

ESSENTIAL OILS TIP

Do not use rosemary oil if you are pregnant and/or nursing, have epilepsy, or are prone to any other seizure disorder or have a fever. You can substitute (same number drops) with orange–*Citrus sinensis* instead. Orange has properties similar to rosemary. Make sure that your orange oil is not oxidized (cloudy) as it will make the skin sensitive. Always keep in a dark bottle, refrigerated, with the cap tightly closed.

20. COFFEE/TOBACCO ADDICTION

It's not unusual for someone addicted to nicotine to be equally addicted to caffeine.

Both nicotine and caffeine are stimulants, especially to the cardiovascular system. Much is demanded of our heart when we introduce these stimulants to our bodies, either separately or together. Nicotine is very addictive and harder to withdraw from than caffeine. Caffeine, in moderation, is actually beneficial to some people.

Aromatherapy can support your resolve in overcoming one or both addictions. Unlike some of the nicotine replacements on the market today, essential oils have no side effects. Everyone feels different when they choose to stop or cut back on either nicotine or caffeine. Some are shaky, nervous, or angry; others feel very weak, lacking energy. The beauty of essential oils is that there is such a variety to choose from, so you can make an individual blend just for you! **Lemon** and **peppermint** will energize you and lift your countenance. **Ylang ylang** and **clary sage** will relax the nervous system, clear negative feelings of anger, help with mental stress, and support deep breathing by opening the diaphragm. Use a dilution rate of 2 percent per 2 tablespoons of carrier.

ENERGIZE ME

6 drops lemon (expands energy outward, uplifts, cleanses)

4 drops peppermint (protects the liver, awakens, supports self-confidence)

CHILL & BREATHE

6 drops clary sage (calms the mind, calms nervous anxiety, supports emotional challenges)

3 drops ylang ylang (nervine, relaxing, supports feelings of joy and pleasure)

MULTIPLE SUPPORT

4 drops clary sage (calms the mind, calms nervous anxiety, supports emotional challenges)

4 drops lemon (or peppermint if you are more drawn to this oil)

4 drops ylang ylang (nervine, relaxing, supports feelings of joy and pleasure)

Use as follows:

Add 4–6 drops in a warm bath. Remember to add the drops *after* you turn off the water and the tub is filled.

Make an inhaler with 15–20 drops of your blend on the wick. Instructions for making an inhaler are found in Section 18. Carry the inhaler with you to inhale when needed.

21. DRUG ADDICTION

This addiction wreaks havoc on the nervous system and liver especially if one has been addicted from a young age. Mentally, the intricate workings of the brain's connections get re-routed. The addict no longer feels worthy of love. Drug addiction is much deeper than a physical challenge—it covers emotional, mental, and spiritual issues as well. Individuals struggling to become free of drug addiction will find the road is not without setbacks. However, aromatherapy can help you gain mental clarity, find relaxation and restful sleep, and gain inner peace and self-worth. Four essential oils to consider are **clary sage, frankincense, lemon,** and **rosemary**.

BREAKING FREE

2 tablespoons of grape seed oil

3 drops clary sage (assists with indecisiveness; calms the nervous system and anxiety)

2 drops lemon (the happy oil; uplifting and cleansing)

3 drops frankincense (quiets the mind bringing focused attention and tranquility)

2 drops rosemary (mild antidepressant property) Note: Omit rosemary if you are pregnant and/or breastfeeding, have epilepsy, are prone to seizures, or have a fever.

Blend oils.

After a shower or bath, put 5–8 drops of blend in your hands. Cup hands over face and inhale 2–3 times, keeping eyes closed. Then, massage blend over entire body.

Before going to bed, massage 3–4 drops of the blend on the bottom of each foot. Feel free to re-apply in the morning upon wakening.

In a 2-ounce plastic spray bottle (PET), add 10–15 drops of the blend first, then 1½ ounces of distilled water and ½ ounce of vegetable glycerin. If you cannot find vegetable glycerin, you can omit it and just use 2 ounces of distilled water. Spray on pillow or where you are resting, or lightly on your face, keeping eyes closed. Shake before each use.

ESSENTIAL OILS TIP

A castor oil pack placed directly over the upper abdomen (directly underneath the breast area) will be an added bonus to the nervous system and liver. You can add 3–4 drops of the Breaking Free blend to the castor oil or just use the castor oil by itself. Directions for how to make a castor oil pack can be found in Section 3.

22. ALCOHOL ADDICTION

You're considered an alcoholic if you're not able to stop drinking, if you function poorly when drinking (and often even when not drinking), and find that recovery time from binge drinking is longer each time. Long-term chronic alcohol use can have a negative impact on every organ and system in the body, from poor coordination, hypertension, and impotence to jaundice, cirrhosis of the liver, and damage to the brain.

Numerous treatments available in communities have been successful. The information here is not intended to replace treatment from physicians and qualified organizations.

How can the use of essential oils support an individual's recovery? Essential oils have energy, and with this energy comes positive emotion. Many people want to stop the pain and suffering they've held at bay with alcohol. **Lemon, peppermint,** and **eucalyptus** can be excellent choices for supporting one's emotional struggles in recovery.

BE FREE

2 tablespoons grape seed oil

3 drops eucalyptus (cleanses negative emotion; clears the mind)

6 drops lemon (outward energy; uplifts and cleanses)

3 drops peppermint (halts suffering; is emotionally uplifting; clears away negative energy)

Thoroughly blend all oils. Use in a bath by adding 3–4 drops after the tub is full. Take the blend with you when you go for a massage.

After a shower use 4–6 drops in an unscented body lotion and massage your whole body.

Inhale the blend as needed during the day to help dispel negative emotions.

Rub 2–3 drops on the bottoms of feet before going to bed, getting up in the morning, or both.

23. ADDICTION WITHDRAWAL

You have chosen your recovery program and are doing well making the journey back to yourself. There are some bumps in the road ahead, but you're confident you can succeed.

Along the way you'll face such challenges as a fuzzy brain (it's hard to put things together mentally); a lack of restful sleep; anxiety; headaches and body aches, and moments of depression or sadness. These challenges are a positive sign of your progress. Do not give up!

Essential oils will support the road to recovery, bringing emotional and physical healing. There are four that deserve consideration: **ginger, lavender, lemon,** and **peppermint**.

JOURNEY BACK TO ME

3 drops ginger (mild stimulant, mood lifting; promotes mental clarity)
3 drops lavender (brings "peace" and
   calm; relaxing; aids in restful sleep)
3 drops lemon (supports good energy and
   lifts negative moods; relieves stress)
3 drops peppermint (helps with minor
   body aches/pains; opens breathing
   airways)

Thoroughly blend all oils.

Use in a bath by adding 3–4 drops after the tub is full. Take the blend with you when you go for a massage.

After a shower use 4–6 drops in an un-scented body lotion and massage the whole body.

Inhale the blend as needed during the day to help dispel negative emotions.

Rub 2–3 drops on the bottoms of the feet before going to bed, getting up in the morning, or both.

ESSENTIAL OILS TIP

If you are pregnant, under a doctor's care or on numerous medications, consult your medical practitioner before using essential oils.

Chapter 2
HORMONES

Sometimes we can't live with them, but always we can't live without them. That's right—hormones. What are they for, anyway? Simply, they are the chemical messengers inside our body that balance organs and systems. In our brain the hypothalamus makes hormones. These are then sent to the pituitary gland and from there they are released through the body to the particular organ or the system in need. If one hormone is not "playing nice" with another hormone, we will know it. We need hormones to function in our daily life and feel good.

If you are stressed, the hypothalamus will send you some cortisol to get a bit more oxygen to the brain while simultaneously releasing energy from glucose and fat. If you ignore your stress and your body has to try to maintain itself, there will be an imbalance of cortisol and you will feel exhausted. To help balance stress in life do some cardio exercise 15–30 minutes a day. Then there is melatonin for some "sweet slumber." At the beginning of evening, when it starts getting dark, melatonin spreads throughout our body. If you sleep with any sort of light, natural or artificial (cell phone, TV, laptop), melatonin has a hard time working. Sleeping in total darkness and without constricting clothing can support the natural release of melatonin so you feel good upon wakening.

These are just two of the numerous hormones we need to stay healthy and feel good. The following chapter will deal with a variety of health issues that can arise from unbalanced hormones and show how we can use essential oils to give our body the nudge needed to keep our hormones balanced. Should you have severe issues with hormonal imbalance, seek proper medical and/or nutritional help from a professional.

24. PMS

The imbalance in hormones days prior to a menstrual cycle will affect the majority of cells in a woman's body. This can result in uncontrollable crying, anger, irritability, depression, concentration problems, tender breasts, weight gain, and headaches. The symptoms and their severity will vary from woman to woman. When this imbalance happens, your family, friends, and even you cannot physically see the imbalance of hormones, only the results of it. Also important to note is that the duration of symptoms also will vary from woman to woman.

Three oils to help address a combination of PMS challenges are **clary sage, geranium,** and **lemon**. The following synergy blend may provide the support you need.

PMS RELIEF

2 tablespoons grape seed oil

5 drops clary sage (hormonal properties for balance; antidepressant, antispasmodic; calms the mind and nerves)

5 drops geranium (assists in regulating hormones; antidepressant, anti-inflammatory)

5 drops lemon (assists with bloating; uplifts and promotes happy feelings)

Use in a bath by adding 3–4 drops after tub is full. After a shower use 4–6 drops in unscented body lotion and massage whole body.

Massage over lower abdomen, hips, and lower back.

Inhale the blend as needed during the day for PMS symptoms.

Rub 2–3 drops on the bottoms of the feet (especially on both sides of your ankles) before going to bed, getting up in the morning, or both.

ESSENTIAL OILS TIP

A good way to know which oils your body may need more of is through inhalation. Inhale each oil one by one. Note how it makes you feel and where you feel it. If you find one oil affects you more than another, decrease the other oils by 1–2 drops and increase your favored oil one drop at a time, inhaling after each drop until the aroma is perfect. Don't forget to write your new recipe down for future blends.

25. IRREGULAR PERIODS

The majority of women will experience irregular periods at some point. This can be caused by pregnancy, stress (too much cortisol interferes with estrogen and progesterone levels), diet (too many unhealthy carbohydrates unbalance hormone production), medications, and excessive exercising (takes energy away from normal hormone production). There are, of course, other reasons, and if you suspect a serious underlying problem, seek medical attention.

For the woman dealing with the challenges of diet, exercise, and stress, here are a few essential oils to the rescue.

A visit with **clary sage, lavender,** and **rosemary** may be of great relief to your body and yourself. Clary sage supports your hormonal health, lavender will support the lessening of anxiety and stress, and rosemary can decrease high levels of cortisol when stress is chronic. We can put them together as follows:

BALANCE

2 tablespoons grape seed oil

5 drops clary sage (properties for hormone balancing; calms the mind and nervous system)

5 drops lavender (antidepressant; calming, nurturing; reduces panic attacks)

5 drops rosemary (decreases high levels of cortisol; energizes and uplifts)

Thoroughly blend all oils together.

Use in a bath by adding 3–4 drops after the tub is full. After a shower use 4–6 drops in unscented body lotion and massage the whole body.

Massage over lower abdomen, hips, and lower back.

Inhale the blend as needed during the day for PMS symptoms.

Rub 2–3 drops on the bottoms of the feet (especially on both sides of your ankles) before going to bed, getting up in the morning, or both.

ESSENTIAL OILS TIP

If you suspect you are pregnant or if you are under a holistic or medical treatment plan, do not use essential oils without discussing it with a professional.

26. INCONTINENCE

Urinary Incontinence (UI) is a loss of bladder control or leakage, meaning urine will leak out of the bladder before you can get to the bathroom. Millions of men and women have this problem either daily or occasionally.

Women can experience UI due to pregnancy, childbirth, or menopause. Both men and women can experience UI due to constipation, medication, caffeine/alcohol, infections, nerve damage, and excess weight. At times, there is pain associated with this condition. There are different types of UI, with physical stress (sneezing, coughing, laughing, exercising) being the most common cause.

Two essential oils that may add support to the treatment of your choice are **ylang ylang** and **lavender**.

UI SUPPORT

2 tablespoons grape seed oil
6 drops lavender (anti-spasmodic, anti-inflammatory; relaxing)
4 drops ylang ylang (anti-inflammatory, relaxing)

Thoroughly blend all oils together.

Apply topically over bladder area on abdomen twice a day. You can also apply topically on the insides of both feet from mid arch down to the heel. Use in a bath by adding 3–4 drops after the tub is full. After a shower use 4–6 drops in unscented body lotion and massage over your whole body.

Inhale when needed.

ESSENTIAL OILS TIP

Kegel exercises strengthen the pelvic muscles. This exercise has helped many people reduce or even cure stress leakage. See your doctor or nurse for correct instructions on how to do this exercise.

27. HEADACHES

Our bodies' hormones fluctuate every day, and when estrogen levels drop this can be the beginning of a headache or a migraine. There are numerous causes for this hormonal fluctuation, including menstruation, pregnancy, hormone replacement therapy, menopause, and sometimes genetics. Other factors that may induce a headache or migraine are skipping a meal, sleep issues (too much or too little), intense lighting or sounds, food sensitivities or allergies, and even the weather.

So, you "feel" the beginnings of a headache, what can you do? Drink water; if you are able to lie down, do so in a dark room where it's quiet; breathe deeply; massage the area of pain; and/or place a cool washcloth over your eyes while lying down. What works for one person may not work for another.

Keep track of what triggers your headaches and address that problem. Sometimes it's helpful to maintain a journal.

For headaches, **peppermint** or **lavender** are the most effective essential oils. Both are analgesic (pain numbing) and offer the calming support that is needed, and so easily too!

HEADACHE RELIEF

3 drops lavender (anti-inflammatory, analgesic, soothing, nurturing)
1 drop peppermint (analgesic, antispasmodic, anti-inflammatory)
2 drops grape seed oil

Massage around the temples, the back of neck (base of the skull), and all around your hairline.

ESSENTIAL OILS TIP

If you are pregnant or think you may be, consult with your holistic or medical practitioner before using essential oils. Peppermint can be a skin irritant, so diluting with a carrier oil is recommended. Do not store peppermint alongside any homeopathic remedies as it may nullify the effectiveness of them. Use a low dilution of peppermint . . . less is more.

28. BREAST PAIN

We enhance them with lacy undergarments. They bring nourishment to our babies. We allow them to be fondled by our lover. And yet, we may ignore them by not touching them monthly for signs of tissue change. Our breasts may even be painful during our monthly changes in estrogen and progesterone, feeling swollen and lumpy. If we are past menopause and taking hormone replacement therapy, we may experience similar breast pain. Sometimes the pain can come simply from our bra not fitting properly or we may have gained some weight.

There are positive actions to consider when dealing with breast pain. Eat clean and organic when possible and include fruits, vegetables, and grains while limiting your salt intake. Wear a bra that not only fits you properly but has excellent support. You may need to reduce caffeine, soft drinks, and chocolate (yes, I'm so sorry, chocolate). Some breast pain stems from stress.

We can also give our breasts some support, nourishment, and comfort. How do **geranium** and **lavender** sound?

BEAUTIFUL BREASTS

2 tablespoons grape seed oil

5 drops geranium (the "woman's oil," balances hormones; anti-inflammatory)

10 drops lavender (analgesic, anti-inflammatory, relaxing)

Thoroughly blend all oils. Massage over entire breast area twice a day.

ESSENTIAL OILS TIP

If you detect a lump in your breast, or one or both are persistently sore, let your doctor know as soon as possible. If you are pregnant and/or breastfeeding, do not use essential oils without first consulting with a holistic or medical practitioner educated in essential oils and who has experience working with pregnant women.

29. IRREGULAR HEARTBEAT

Out of nowhere you feel a flutter. Your heart is pounding in your chest, your pulse increases, you feel lightheaded, weak, and a bit anxious. What just happened? For many women challenged with menopause, when your estrogen level changes, irregular heartbeats begin.

Estrogen is an important hormone for a woman's overall health, inclusive of her heart. When these levels begin dropping, your sympathetic nervous system will get overstimulated and result in an irregular heartbeat. Other causes may be an overactive thyroid, medication, low oxygen levels in your blood, or anemia. In addition, there's anxiety, exercise, caffeine, nicotine, and diet pills. So, if you are experiencing irregular heartbeats in excess and they are accompanied by chest pain, sweating, and/or shortness of breath, do not delay in seeking medical attention.

The following essential oils will be helpful for when the heartbeat is irregular and you want immediate support: **lavender** and **ylang ylang**.

BE CALM MY HEART

2 tablespoons grape seed oil

3 drops lavender (sedative, calming)

1 drop ylang ylang (sedative will help slow rapid heart palpitations)

Thoroughly blend all oils. Massage clockwise over the chest area during irregular heartbeat. Inhale the blend.

ESSENTIAL OILS TIP

Ylang ylang may lower blood pressure. If you already live with low blood pressure do not use ylang ylang. Substitute two drops of geranium, as it supports the regulating of hormones and encourages calmness.

30. DIZZINESS

Have you experienced feelings of dizziness? It's not uncommon. At the least it can be annoying; at most it may be a symptom of something more serious. There are numerous reasons for dizziness such as fatigue, motion sickness, vertigo, medications, hypoglycemia (low blood sugar), and menopause. If you are having dizzy spells more often than not, it is advisable to seek medical attention as soon as possible.

Here we're mainly concerned with the dizziness that comes with a woman's journey through menopause. Lots of changes are happening internally and externally. A woman's hormones are changing and estrogen is declining. Some positive actions to take if you experience dizziness are:

- Drink plenty of water.
- Exercise daily for 20–30 minutes.
- Make sure you're getting restorative sleep.
- Stop smoking.
- Reduce alcohol intake.
- Take warm showers.

Essential oils that may bring relief are **lavender, peppermint,** and **rosemary**. Let's make a blend.

BE STILL

2 tablespoons grape seed oil
4 drops lavender (sedative, calming)
3 drops peppermint (stimulant)
3 drops rosemary (stimulant)

Thoroughly blend all oils. Apply topically to the forehead, temples, and near the outer ear as needed.

ESSENTIAL OILS TIP

Do not use rosemary oil if you are pregnant and/or breastfeeding, have epilepsy, are prone to seizures, or have a fever. In any of these cases, omit rosemary and substitute two drops of ginger.

31. OSTEOPOROSIS

We have an amazing substance living inside us that busily replaces itself about every ten years! Bone. If you are low on calcium, vitamin D, estrogen, or if there is family history of bone loss, you should be proactive in maintaining healthy bones. There are, of course, other factors that contribute to bone loss such as smoking, abusing alcohol, or having a low body weight. Unfortunately, there are no warning signs of osteoporosis. If you notice you are "shrinking" and/or "hunching over," have unexplained spinal pain, or your bones fracture easily, you should seek medical support.

If you are diagnosed with osteoporosis, a variety of treatments are available One of the best treatments is exercise. Both cardio and weight training are important to support the health of the bones and perhaps even encourage the re-growth of lost bone.

There's a blend of essential oils to support bone health, relax you, and relieve pain. They are **clove, geranium, ginger,** and **peppermint**.

BEAUTIFUL BONES

2 tablespoons grape seed oil

2 drops clove (warming, analgesic— numbs pain)

4 drops geranium (regulates hormones; anti-inflammatory)

3 drops ginger (analgesic, anti-inflammatory)

1 drop peppermint (analgesic, uplifting)

Thoroughly blend all oils. Use 4 drops of the blend in a warm bath, making sure the tub is full and the water is turned off before adding the blend.

Massage the blend directly onto the joints that are affected.

32. VAGINAL DRYNESS

As a woman's supply and quality of her eggs decrease, so, too, does the hormone estrogen. Eventually this journey takes her to the menopausal and postmenopausal years.

The drop in estrogen may cause your vaginal lining to become thin, resulting in dryness, itching, and irritation. You may also be more susceptible to vaginal infections at this time. Vaginal dryness at times also may be due to medications, diabetes, or sexually transmitted diseases. If you are experiencing pain, bleeding, or unusual discharge, seek medical attention.

To help lubricate the vaginal lining, include more healthy fat like flax seed in your diet. Also, instead of having coffee or soda, choose water or your favorite broth. Exercise geared toward strengthening the pelvic floor and toning vaginal tissues may help.

The essential oils **frankincense** and **lavender** will soothe mucus membranes and are anti-inflammatory. This recipe is a 1 percent dilution.

VAGINAL HEALTH

2 tablespoons of organic vegetable glycerin (makes essential oils less harmful)
2 drops frankincense (soothes mucus membranes)
2 drops lavender (anti-inflammatory; soothes vaginal tissue)

Thoroughly blend all ingredients. Add 4 drops of blend to a sitz bath by letting your bathtub fill to hip level. Soak in the tub for 10–15 minutes.

Make a cream by adding 2–3 drops of blend to 3 ounces of your favorite vaginal lubricant on the market.

ESSENTIAL OILS TIP

If you find these essential oils to be too aggressive, then they are not for you. Many homeopathic remedies also work very well. The key is to explore the natural and medicinal help available and make your own choice.

33. MOOD SWINGS

You love to swing. The motion of back and forth in the air is exhilarating—except if it is your mood that is swinging. You're happy, you're sad . . . you're angry, you're glad! When your hormones begin to swing, so does your state of mind. It happens to everyone, and your mood can change without notice. When your mood is upbeat you're a pleasure to be with. A troublesome mood will quickly bring you down.

Inhaling essential oils can support you through the troublesome moods. The following oils can help with the pendulum of emotions:

- **Clary sage** (brings hormonal balance for PMS related emotions)
- **Frankincense** (calms anxiety and nervousness)
- **Geranium** (brings hormonal balance for PMS related emotions)
- **Lavender** (calms insecurity)
- **Peppermint** (gives energy when you are feeling sluggish or slow)
- **Rosemary** (energizing and uplifting) Do not use if you are pregnant and/or nursing, have epilepsy, a fever, or are prone to seizures.
- **Ylang ylang** (calms anger and frustration)

After you find the oil(s) that you may need, simply add 2–3 drops onto a cotton ball and inhale deeply 3–4 times. You can also take a warm bath, and after filling the tub, turn off the water and add 3 drops of your chosen oil to the water. *Note:* Don't use peppermint in the bath, as it can be a skin irritant, and that would not help your mood!

ESSENTIAL OILS TIP

If you find that your mood swings are severe or nothing seems to help, the suggestions presented in this chapter are not a substitute or a replacement for professional medical help.

34. FATIGUE

"I'm so tired." Does this sound familiar? Fatigue can creep up on you. There are so many responsibilities and daily challenges in life now. Excess emotional stress, depression, hormonal imbalance, and poor food choices can all cause fatigue.

Some positive changes to your life will get some energy back: Start by getting restorative sleep. Be sure not to have any stimulating food or beverage, or exercise two to three hours before you go to bed. Exercise is very important for fatigue, especially walking each day, but it is better not to exercise near bedtime. Last, but not least, give back to yourself. Create time for the activities that you enjoy.

Essential oils can help you feel invigorated, alert, and restful. Essential oils proven to help with fatigue are:

- **Eucalyptus** (analgesic—pain relieving; stimulating; clears the mind for focusing)
- **Geranium** (balances hormones; uplifting; relieves stress)
- **Lemon** (the "happy" oil, full of outward and expanding energy)
- **Peppermint** (analgesic, stimulating for the mind; supports self-confidence)

- **Rosemary** (aids memory; stimulating; clears negative thoughts)

Inhale the oils for immediate refreshment. Put 2–3 drops of your favorite oil on a cotton ball, place in zip lock bag, and take with you to **inhale** as needed throughout the day.

ENERGIZING

2 drops eucalyptus

4 drops geranium

3 drops lemon

2 drops peppermint

4 drops rosemary

Blend all the oils.

After a warm bath or shower, add the oil blend to 2 tablespoons of unscented body lotion and massage all over your body.

ESSENTIAL OILS TIP

If you find this blend too stimulating to use before bed, omit the rosemary and geranium. If you are using peppermint oil, be sure to keep it away from any homeopathic products as it could cause them to become ineffective. If you are pregnant and/or breastfeeding, have epilepsy, a fever, or are prone to seizures, do not use rosemary.

35. EXHAUSTION

Fatigue, left untreated, leads to mental, physical, and emotional exhaustion. This will pose extremely serious health challenges such as high or low blood pressure, ulcers, bowel issues, and breathing challenges. When you become exhausted the slightest thing makes you feel like you will explode . . . and you just might.

Using essential oils in your recovery can be an immense support. Here is a recipe using **clary sage, frankincense, and lavender**.

TIME FOR ME . . . BLEND 1

2 tablespoons grape seed oil

5 drops clary sage (calms the mind and eases nervous anxiety; supports emotional challenges)

5 drops frankincense (supports nervous system; calms the mind; assists with tranquility)

6 drops lavender (antidepressant, calming, soothing; reduces anxiety and fear; calms panic attacks; brings balance to all body systems)

Thoroughly blend all oils together. Massage all over your body especially before going to bed. Apply a few drops on the bottoms of both feet at bedtime.

After using this blend, make this next blend, **Time for Me . . . Blend 2**, by adding 2 drops of lemon (the "happy" oil, expanding energy) to Blend 1. Continue to use your first blend at night but now begin to use Blend 2 in the mornings.

ESSENTIAL OILS TIP

You can place a castor oil pack on the core of your abdomen (right under the breast area). If you want, add 2 drops of Blend 1 to the castor oil. Refer back to Section 3.

36. NIGHT SWEATS OR HOT FLASHES

There you are just going about your daily routine or you are in a peaceful slumber and out of nowhere a sudden and intense heat rushes into your upper body and face! The heat continues for seconds but it feels likes hours. If you are pre-menopausal or menopausal, the fluctuating of estrogen and progesterone has just confused your poor hypothalamus into sending out signals that affect heat-inducing circulation.

Essential oils are a wonderful addition to a woman's arsenal during menopause for the therapeutic properties of the oils that balance hormones and cool the body at the same time. Put together this quick recipe consisting of **clary sage, geranium, lemon,** and **peppermint**.

Apply a few drops to the big toe of each foot.

After filling a bathtub with warm water and turning off the faucet, add 3–5 drops of the blend to the water and relax for 15–20 minutes.

Make a spray in a 2-ounce plastic (PET) bottle by adding 15 drops of the blend first and then 1½ ounces of distilled water and ½ ounce of vegetable glycerin. Store in the refrigerator. Use immediately when hot flashes start. Shake well before using.

Inhale the blend when needed.

COOLING DOWN

2 tablespoons grape seed oil

6 drops clary sage (hormone balancing)

5 drops geranium (hormone balancing, cooling)

3 drops lemon (uplifting)

2 drops peppermint (febrifuge—fever reducing; uplifting)

Thoroughly blend all oils.

Massage all over your body.

37. LOSS OF LIBIDO

For men, it's usually erectile dysfunction. For women, it can be both mental and/or physical. Reasons for women can include stress, poor body image, depression, unbalanced hormones, painful intercourse, and fatigue. It is wise to seek medical and/or integrative support at this time.

Essential oils help with the normal ups and downs of libido in a woman's life. Remembering that the home of sexual desire is the limbic system of our brain (inhalation), let's make a blend using: **clary sage, ginger, geranium, and ylang ylang**.

HELLO LIBIDO

2 tablespoons grape seed oil

5 drops clary sage (female tonic; boosts sexual confidence)

3 drops ginger (warming; combats burnout)

3 drops grapefruit (refreshes, energizes)

3 drops ylang ylang (promotes sensual awareness; relaxing)

Thoroughly blend all oils.

Add 3–5 drops of the blend to a bath and soak for 15 minutes. Add 4–6 drops of the blend to your body lotion and massage (or have your special someone massage) it all over your body.

Make a pillow spray in a 2-ounce plastic (PET) bottle by first adding 12–15 drops of the blend, followed by 1½ ounces distilled water, and ½ ounce vodka. Spray on bedding.

Inhale the blend.

JASMINE AND ROSE

Jasmine absolute–*Jasminum grandiflorum* and rose absolute–*Rosa damascena* are two other choices. Absolutes have a thicker consistency. Allow them to warm to room temperature before using. Both jasmine and rose are very sensual. When using jasmine, only use 1 drop per 2 tablespoons of carrier oil; do not use jasmine if you are pregnant or breastfeeding, and do not use it on a prolonged basis. You can use up to 3 drops of rose per 2 tablespoons of carrier. Both jasmine and rose are very expensive, but you will use only drops at a time and if you keep them stored properly they will last for years. They are worth the investment.

38. SLEEP . . . INSOMNIA

"Oh, sweet slumber, where art thou?" Sleep is such a needed gift. If needed sleep is escaping us, then it may be time to look at our habits.

Coffee and tea are stimulants, especially if we indulge in them before going to bed. Stress is another culprit. If you are dieting, are you really getting enough food and nutrients? Are you so tired or fatigued that you can't sleep? Perhaps your hormones are creating some challenges. If you see yourself in any of these situations, do the best to make some changes. If sleep is eluding you for other reasons, seek professional medical and/or integrative support.

The essential oils that may help are **clary sage, lavender,** and **ylang ylang**. The combination of therapeutic properties will include hormonal balancing, calming, pain relieving and having a sedative effect. You can make the following blend to use before you go to bed:

SWEET SLUMBER

2 tablespoons grape seed oil

4 drops clary sage (hormone balancing; calming)

6 drops lavender (analgesic—pain numbing; calming, soothing)

2 drops ylang ylang (analgesic, sedative, relaxing)

Thoroughly blend all oils.

Add 2–3 drops of the blend to your unscented body lotion and massage your body.

Add 2–3 drops of the blend to a warm bath after you have turned off the water. Do not add more than 3 drops to the bath water as you do not want to fall asleep in the tub.

Rub 2–3 drops of the blend on the bottoms of both feet before going to bed.

39. POOR CONCENTRATION

Have you ever played the game Concentration? If you want to win you have to devote all your attention and stay mentally focused. Could you play it now? If not, don't feel bad. The amount of stress in today's environment affects all of us at one time or another.

There are times, however, when we need some support. Maybe you're writing a book, or have a long day of business meetings, or you need to help your children with school projects. Whatever your circumstances, essential oils can be just the friend your brain needs.

Let's see what oils from this book can help:

- **Clary sage** (stimulates creativity; supports emotional and energetic challenges)
- **Clove** (increases energy; warming; enhances alertness)
- **Lemon** (uplifts and cleanses; increases creativity)
- **Peppermint** (awakens; clears energy; uplifts; stimulates creativity)
- **Rosemary** (boosts alertness; encourages clarity; strengthens the mind) Do not use if you are epileptic, prone to seizures, pregnant, and/or breastfeeding.

You can use any single oil or put them together in a synergy blend as follows:

ATTENTION

3 drops clary sage

2 drops lemon

1 drop peppermint

3 drops rosemary

Thoroughly blend all oils together.

One of the easiest ways to use this blend is by diffusing it. If you do not have a diffuser, then use your stove and a cooking pot. Fill the pot with 2 cups of water, heat the water until right before the boiling point, turn off the heat, and add 3 drops of a single oil or 3 drops of your blend.

ESSENTIAL OILS TIP

There are a variety of diffusers on the market today. There are nebulizing, humidifying, heat, and evaporating diffusers that distribute the oils into the air differently. Some are electric, some are burners. If you have an aromatherapist in your area stop in and seek her or his thoughts. If not, do some research online. If you choose one with a glass holder for oils it will get messy, but the ones with pads or that allow you to add water are wonderful.

40. BAD MEMORY

Have you ever gone to your kitchen, stopped dead in your tracks and thought really, really hard about what you came there for? The good news is that it happens to just about everyone. We all experience lapses in memory.

Usually this is because we've got way too much on our plate. We're juggling so many responsibilities that our brain just takes a time out. How can essential oils help? The inhalation of oils goes directly to the limbic system. From there the brain signals where in your body the volatile molecules are needed. At the same time, your lungs accept the volatile molecules and pass them into your bloodstream! Aren't you happy we don't have to remember to tell our brain and lungs to do this?

Oils that will help memory are:

- **Ginger** (combats burnout; stimulates energy)
- **Geranium** (opens up the sensory world; helps with concentration)
- **Lavender** (nurtures; calms the mind)
- **Peppermint** (wakes up the mind)
- **Rosemary** (stimulates the brain; enhances memory) Do not use if you are epileptic, prone to seizures, pregnant, and/or breastfeeding.

As with concentration, the best use of the oils is inhalation or diffusing into the air. You can try the following recipe or make your own using the oil(s) you are drawn to:

BRAIN FOG-GONE

2 drops ginger

4 drops geranium

6 drops lavender

3 drops peppermint (Store separately from homeopathic remedies, as peppermint may weaken their effectiveness.)

2 drops rosemary (Omit if you are pregnant and/or breastfeeding, have epilepsy, a fever, or are prone to seizures.)

Thoroughly blend all the oils together.

If you do not have a diffuser, then use your stove and a cooking pot. Fill pot with 2 cups of water, heat the water until right before the boiling point, turn off the heat and add 3 drops of a single oil or 3 drops of your blend. The uplifting scent will permeate your home, or you can bring the water mixture into the room where you need it and let the oils evaporate, and enjoy! For information on purchasing a diffuser see Section 39.

41. ENDOMETRIOSIS

Endometrial cells are supposed to line the inside of the uterus, pelvis, and other areas. Why these cells decide to grow outside of the uterus is not known. Not only is this extremely painful during menstruation and sexual intimacy, it may prevent pregnancy. The earlier it is diagnosed the better, usually through laparoscopy.

Endometriosis affects the woman's body and her emotions. Prescribed drugs have side effects such as hot flashes, sweating, weight gain, skin challenges, and nervousness. Some women look for more integrative therapy to help with the pain, inflammation, and spasms that accompany endometriosis.

Use of essential oils addresses both physical and emotional challenges that come with endometriosis. Some oils to consider are:

- **Clary sage** (balances hormones; antispasmodic; calms nervous anxiety)
- **Frankincense** (analgesic—numbs pain; anti-inflammatory; encourages tranquility)
- **Geranium** (balances hormones; anti-inflammatory; antispasmodic)
- **Lavender** (anti-inflammatory; sedative; analgesic; nurturing; calming)

To make a massage blend you can use the following:

"END"OMETRIOSIS

2 tablespoons grape seed oil
2 drops clary sage
2 drops frankincense
2 drops geranium
4 drops lavender

Thoroughly blend all the oils.

Massage gently over hip and lower abdomen up to 3 times a day when pain is present.

Prepare a castor oil pack and add 4 drops of the blend to the castor oil. Directions for a castor oil pack are in Section 3.

42. EDEMA

We may inherit this condition, indulge in too much sodium, be pregnant, sit in one position too long, have just been injured, or are taking a medication. Whatever the reason, excess fluid is leaking from our capillaries and building up in the surrounding tissue. We are left with swollen hands, feet, and/or arms.

Some women drink nettle or dandelion tea to assist the body as a natural diuretic. It may be good to also have a balanced sodium intake while eliminating the excess fluid. You can find relief by lying down with your feet elevated higher than your heart.

Additionally, you can make the following blend of essential oils to give support and bring relief:

EDEMA SUPPORT

2 tablespoons grape seed oil

4 drops ginger (diaphoretic—promotes perspiration and elimination through skin; anti-inflammatory)

6 drops lavender (anti-inflammatory; analgesic—pain reducer; balances all body systems)

Thoroughly blend all oils.

Massage your feet and legs, hands and arms and lower back as follows: With edema massage, always move toward the heart, i.e., start at feet and move *up* the leg toward the heart; start at the fingers and move toward the heart *up* the arm; on the back (not abdomen) move from top of buttocks *up* toward heart. Do once per day until excess fluid is gone.

ESSENTIAL OILS TIP

This chapter is not about Lymphedema or Lipedema, which are extremely serious conditions that need medical and/or integrative support. If your edema is long lasting and you experience chest pain, dizziness, and/or shortness of breath, seek appropriate attention. If you are pregnant and/or breastfeeding, consult a certified aromatherapist and/or medical professional with essential oil training before using essential oils.

43. LOW ENERGY

It's like when your car won't start and some nice person gives you a jump. That's how we feel from time to time when we lack energy . . . we need a "jump start." When our body and brain become slackers, essential oils can come to the rescue! Let's take 3 from the book:

- **Ginger** (gives life to the nervous system; aids in restorative sleep)
- **Peppermint** (stimulating; calming to the nervous system)
- **Rosemary** (stimulant; tonic for low energy and mental fatigue)

Let's make a blend:

JUMP START

2 tablespoons grape seed oil

6 drops ginger

2 drops peppermint

2 drops rosemary (Do not use if you are pregnant and/or breastfeeding, have epilepsy, a fever, or are prone to seizures.)

Thoroughly blend all oils.

After a shower or bath, massage the oil blend over your body. Use 3–4 drops of the blend on the bottoms of feet before going to bed.

You can also inhale the oils individually. Place 3–4 drops on a cotton ball and inhale as needed. You can place the cotton ball in a plastic zipper bag to carry with you.

44. FIBROMYALGIA

"It's all in your head," says the doctor. "Yes," you say, "and in my back and legs and neck and spine!" Then, there is the fatigue, stiffness, depression, memory lapse, and sleeplessness that partners with the pain. Fibromyalgia is not well understood. Hormones are known to be related to the condition. Sleep is imperative, so getting a good night's rest will help. Essential oils can also assist in alleviating pain and inflammation, and inducing sleep. Let's work with **lavender, peppermint, rosemary,** and **ylang ylang** to see how they will help in a synergy blend.

FIBRO-OUTTA-MY-WAY

2 tablespoons grape seed oil

3 drops lavender (analgesic—numbs pain; antidepressant; anti-inflammatory; nurturing)

2 drops peppermint (analgesic; anti-inflammatory; cooling; uplifting)

3 drops rosemary (antispasmodic; analgesic; nourishes nervous system; uplifting) Do not use if you are pregnant and/or breastfeeding, have epilepsy, a fever, or are prone to seizures.

3 drops ylang ylang (analgesic; anti-inflammatory; nervine; sedative; relaxing)

Thoroughly blend all oils.

For a compress: In one cup of water add 8 drops of blend. Put a small cloth in the cup to absorb the mixture and place on the point of pain. You can use either hot or cold water, depending on which works better. Use this treatment as often as you may need it.

Bath: After filling the tub and shutting off the water, massage a small amount on your painful areas and then sit in the warm bath 15–30 minutes.

Massage: Take the blend with you to get a full body massage or use yourself over your body. Make sure to use some on the bottoms of your feet.

45. INFLAMMATION

There are many causes of inflammation: unbalanced hormones, injury, illness, chemicals, and even the food we eat. Usually there is swelling, pain; sometimes redness and heat. Often when one part of the body is inflamed, another part gets inflamed to help out. If you hurt your leg and ignore it, then your hip and other leg will begin to compensate for the injured leg. This is added inflammation your body must cope with, and in time, (if ignored) your posture will become affected as well as other systems. This will place great stress and inflammation on the nervous system. With your nerves now dealing with extra inflammation at the expense of balancing other parts of your body, you will begin to feel sick. Thus, a large part of the body can become inflamed.

A considerable number of essential oils have anti-inflammatory properties. What are also needed are oils that contain therapeutic properties for pain and swelling, and oils that bring nourishment to the nervous system. **Clove, frankincense, peppermint,** and **rosemary** may prove to be helpful in dealing with inflammation.

INFLAMMATION RESCUE

2 tablespoons grape seed oil

2 drops clove (warm, analgesic—numbs pain; relieves swelling)

3 drops frankincense (strengthens immune system; analgesic; anti-inflammatory)

2 drops peppermint (analgesic; antispasmodic; anti-inflammatory; cooling

3 drops rosemary (antispasmodic; analgesic)

Thoroughly blend all oils.

Add 5–6 drops of the blend to your unscented body lotion and massage your body after a shower or bath. Apply 3–4 drops of the blend to the bottoms of your feet before going to bed. Put 4–5 drops of the blend on a cotton ball to inhale when needed.

ESSENTIAL OILS TIP

If you are pregnant and/or breastfeeding, have epilepsy, a fever, or are prone to seizures do not use rosemary. You can substitute 3 drops of lavender.

Store peppermint away from homeopathic remedies as it may nullify their effectiveness.

46. JET LAG

When our internal clock gets out of synchronization because of traveling through or visiting different time zones, whether across the country or halfway around the world, we may have several days of dreariness until our internal clock catches up to our new environment.

Here's a plan of attack for the future so as not to miss out on any beautiful scenery and/or experiences abroad. Use **peppermint** and **eucalyptus** before and during traveling.

Make an **inhaler** (see Section 18) using 6 drops of peppermint and 5 drops of eucalyptus. Upon arriving at your destination, continue using the inhaler to stay awake until the local time for bed comes.

At bedtime, add 2 drops of **lavender** and 1 drop of **geranium** to a warm bath. If you shower, add those drops to your unscented body lotion and massage over your body and on the bottoms of your feet, after your shower.

Upon awakening, use your inhaler and at end of day your bath or shower blend. Continue until you feel your body in the "groove" with your destination. To adapt more easily when you return from the trip, use the same method.

ESSENTIAL OILS TIP

Grapefruit–*Citrus x paradisi* is worthy of mention; consider adding 3 drops to your inhaler. This is an excellent oil for relieving fatigue. Caution: If you are on medications, check with your doctor or pharmacist first, as grapefruit oil can be a contraindication for some medications. Also, keep your inhaler separate from any homeopathic remedies as the peppermint may nullify their effectiveness.

47. VARICOSE VEINS

Once upon a time our circulatory system would make a marvelous journey every day, from heart to feet to head to heart again. Then one day, we began to wear shoes that were too high or tight, stand on concrete or blacktop, sit all day long at a desk, wear very tight clothing or girdles, gain weight, get pregnant, and so on. We restricted this marvelous journey. Blood flow begins slowing down. Our blood vessels accepted the extra blood. To accommodate the excess, they had to stretch, causing them to weaken. This is the story behind spider and varicose veins.

How can we help our body through this? One important remedy is to elevate your legs when possible, bringing relief to the muscles and blood vessels. Another is to do a very gentle massage of the delicate vessels. Let's use the essential oils of **frankincense, geranium,** and **lavender**.

NOURISHMENT IN VEIN

2 ounces grape seed oil

4 drops frankincense (analgesic—numbs pain; cicatrisant—rejuvenates cells; anti-inflammatory)

2 drops geranium (anti-inflammatory, cooling, antispasmodic)

4 drops lavender (analgesic, anti-inflammatory)

Thoroughly blend all oils.

Gently massage the blend directly over veins in an upward motion. If you want to massage from your foot to your knee do so very gently and always upward toward the heart. You need to support the circulatory system, to move back up the leg. Do not push deep into the leg.

ESSENTIAL OILS TIP

This is not intended to take the place of medical attention, since varicose veins may rupture, causing other problems.

PART 2

WELLBEING

Chapter 3
EMOTIONAL WELLNESS

Our emotions have a profound effect on our body. You may feel you are handling stress, but how in tune are you with the interplay between your feelings and your body? Instead of accepting how we feel, we may deny our feelings by staying so busy there is no time to "feel" them. In turn, we unconsciously demand that our body deal with stress, as well.

How does our emotional health affect us physically?

- The feelings of grief and sorrow are sent to the lungs and colon.
- The feelings of fear are sent to the kidneys and bladder.
- The feelings of anger, resentment, and jealousy are sent to the liver and gallbladder.
- The feelings of everyday stress are sent to the stomach, spleen, and pancreas.
- The feelings of sadness are sent to the heart and small intestine.

The next time you cry, taste your tears. They will be sweet if you cry "happy," salty if you cry "sad," and bitter if you cry "angry." When you cry, your body is immediately addressing the emotion behind the tears. The brain begins to release hormones, directed specifically at the system inundated with the emotion, to bring a balance. That is why after you let yourself have a really good cry, you may feel tired, but you also will feel calm. Tears help us deal with our emotions.

When we hold in our emotions, we allow damage to pile up in the particular system responsible for the emotion. In time, if we have not dealt with our feelings, the overflow will envelope the next system. It's a domino effect. The bottom line is that any emotion we continue to deny will eventually show up to be physically dealt with. The suppressed emotion will cause stress, and stress is at the root of many diseases.

Essential oils for emotional challenges will not cure the underlying issue but will provide comfort, which in turn allows both physical and emotional support. Essential oils have energetic qualities that compensate and fill in what may have gotten lost; they bring balance back. As we continue using the essential oils from this book, we will be able to support our emotions in a healthy direction.

48. DEPRESSION

Sadness and depression at times become intertwined. However, they aren't the same thing. Everyone is sad at different times and for different reasons. Sadness may last a few hours or days. Depression, though, claims your life all day long. Depression turned inward becomes anger. Along with it can come a decline in energy, weight gain, aches and pains, and other symptoms. When depression becomes overwhelming and/or disabling, seek professional help.

Let's put our olfactory region to work and stimulate our limbic system to bring an immediate uplifting refreshment using the oils of **clary sage, frankincense, lemon,** and **lavender**.

UPLIFT AND REFRESH

2 tablespoons grape seed oil

2 drops clary sage (moves stagnant energy; supports emotional challenges; calms the mind)

2 drops frankincense (brings focused attention and tranquility; supports all levels of emotional healing)

2 drops lemon (promotes outward energy)

2 drops lavender (calms, nurtures; reduces anxiety and fear; balances all body systems)

Thoroughly blend all oils.

After a shower or bath massage over your entire body. Add 2–3 drops and apply to the bottom of each foot before bed.

Make an inhaler by placing 2–3 drops of your favorite essential oil on a cotton ball. Put in a zip lock bag to take with you if traveling. Inhale when needed.

ESSENTIAL OILS TIP

If you are under medical supervision or are pregnant and/or breastfeeding, consult with a medical and/or integrative professional for guidance in using these oils safely.

49. NEGATIVITY

Don't allow negativity to clutter your mind. That is easier said than done especially when we have family, friends, or coworkers who seem to thrive on negativity and pessimism. For some people, and maybe you, nothing good comes from anything.

Setting healthy boundaries for yourself is a good starting point. Boundaries are not negative because they will be your "barrier" to keep separate from the ever-draining emotion of negativity coming from others.

Do your best not to take things personally, even if they appear personal. More than likely there are things happening behind the scenes that have nothing to do with you. Showing human kindness will make both you and others feel happy. We are affected by our surroundings, so surround yourself with as many positive people as possible. See how many positive solutions you can come up with in a negative situation. Grow with life's journey of ups and downs. Embrace and learn from both. As hard as it is, do your best not to allow past negative experiences be a thief of your happiness. Each and every new day is *your* gift to cherish.

The essential oils of **frankincense, lavender, lemon,** and **peppermint** can be positive friends. You can make the following blend or choose 1–2 of your favorites and introduce them to each other!

CONTENTMENT

2 tablespoons grape seed oil

3 drops frankincense (energy healing; brings tranquility; quiets the mind)

5 drops lavender (calming, soothing, balancing)

2 drops lemon (simultaneously uplifting and cleansing)

2 drops peppermint (uplifting, awakening; clears stagnate energy; stimulates creativity) Store peppermint away from homeopathic remedies as it may nullify their effectiveness.

Thoroughly blend all oils.

Use as an all over body massage after a shower or bath.

Put 5–6 drops of the blend in a diffuser and place next to you or in a room with company. Make an easy inhaler by placing 2–3 drops of blend on a cotton ball. Inhale when needed.

50. JEALOUSY

There is a healthy jealousy and a very unhealthy one. A healthy jealousy is sincerely guarding what belongs to you against danger. An unhealthy jealousy often stems from a heart that has been hurt. What follows such an injury is loneliness, self-condemnation, a greediness for love; fear, longing, and envy. At the core is a lack of self-love.

If you have no self-love, you will lack the capability to accept love. As desperately as you want to be loved and wanted, you can create a barrier against any further hurt and will never trust again. Ironically, this unhealthy jealousy demands that others love us and trust us, while we don't even love or trust ourselves.

Building a balanced love of yourself takes time but is worth the effort. The oils **eucalyptus, geranium, lavender, peppermint,** and **ylang ylang** can be on your self-love team, easing heartache, balancing emotions, and teaching you how to "breathe."

I LOVE ME

2 tablespoons grape seed oil

1 drop eucalyptus (eases breathing)

4 drops geranium (balances love; encourages self-love)

4 drops lavender (eases heartache; nurtures, soothes)

1 drop peppermint (eases breathing; uplifting)

1 drop ylang ylang (balances the heart; eases heartache; relaxing)

Thoroughly blend all oils.

Add 5–6 drops to unscented body lotion and massage all over your body. Apply 4–5 drops over the chest area in a circular motion at night before bed.

51. IRRITABILITY

It's been a long day. There's another impossible deadline at work. All areas of life are demanding your attention, and you feel like a Gumby doll. Finally, the lid pops off, and all your stored-up irritability comes spilling out like a boiling pot of water.

This can happen to the most even-tempered person. There are also serious and heart wrenching events that happen in life. The death of a loved one. The loss of employment. Long-term illness of yourself or a family member. These will each take a toll; together they add up to irritability.

Essential oils can bring a much-needed calm. They can nurture frayed emotions and balance the mind, body and spirit. Keep your **lavender** within easy reach. Apply 1–2 drops in your hands, cup your face, and breathe deeply. Use on the base of your neck and around your ears. Apply one drop and massage over your chest. Then take a warm bath.

52. HYSTERIA

Hysteria is both a mental and nervous disorder. The afflicted individual may laugh or cry uncontrollably for no reason, find breathing extremely difficult, experience pain in their arms or legs, and suffer loss of consciousness. Emotionally, if you experience hysteria, you may become very insecure and have an intense desire to be loved.

Herbs and supplements have had very favorable results in treating this condition. Adding fruits, vegetables and grains to your diet, along with completely eliminating smoking, white sugar, caffeine, and alcohol have proven to be very promising.

Essential oils can be used in a preventive way but will not of themselves cure hysteria. We will use **clary sage, lavender, peppermint, and ylang ylang**.

CALM ME

2 tablespoons grape seed oil

4 drops clary sage (balances hormones; calms the mind; calms nervous anxiety; supports emotional challenges)

4 drops lavender (antidepressant, calming, nurturing; reduces anxiety and fear)

2 drops ylang ylang (antidepressant, anti-inflammatory; sedative, nervine)

1 drop peppermint (uplifts; encourages open breathing)

Thoroughly blend all oils.

After a shower or bath, put 6–8 drops of the blend in your hands and cup over your face to inhale deeply. Then, massage over your entire body.

Apply 3–4 drops to the bottom of each foot before bed. Inhale the blend as needed.

ESSENTIAL OILS TIP

If you are challenged with hysteria, seek medical and/or integrative support. There are many alternative and natural treatments available. Store your blend separately, due to the peppermint in it, to avoid nullifying any homeopathic remedy you may have.

53. PANIC ATTACKS

You can be anywhere when out of the blue you are suddenly overwhelmed with panic, anxiety, and fear. Your heart feels as if it will burst right out of your chest. Your breathing is sharp and short. You feel dizzy and nauseated, and you're sweating. You feel as if you are detaching from life; going crazy, losing control, and afraid of dying. You're having a panic attack.

Some people regularly experience such attacks. If you're one of them, pay close attention to what triggers the attack. Are you afraid of heights, long bridges, speaking in public, or something similar? These are specific experiences that can set off an attack.

To counter this, we have in our essential oil arsenal **frankincense, lavender,** and **ylang ylang** to help us breathe, boost our mood, and encourage tranquility.

PEACEFUL TRANQUILITY

1 cup Epsom Salts

3 drops frankincense (quiets the mind; brings focused attention and tranquility)

6 drops lavender (calming, nurturing; reduces anxiety and panic attacks)

1 drop ylang ylang (sedative and nervine)

Thoroughly blend all the oils.

Pour Epsom Salts directly under running water in the bathtub. When the tub is full, turn off the water and add 4 drops of the blend to the water. Soak in the warm bath for 20–30 minutes. Relax.

ESSENTIAL OILS TIP

If you have a panic attack, use one to two drops of lavender. Apply the oil "neat," without a carrier, directly over the chest, at the base of the neck and around the ears. Inhale the oil.

54. A LACK OF GROUNDING

It's great to fly—to soar, in fact. But sooner or later you have to come back to reality. If you don't, if you consistently refuse to reconnect with the real world, you're potentially headed for disaster. If you have trouble returning to earth, try one of these:

- Take your shoes off and walk barefoot! If you live by a beach, walk in the sand and let the ocean talk to you. You will exfoliate your feet, mind, and spirit. If you live somewhere else, walk in your backyard (where it is safe), or find a tranquil spot in your area to visit.
- Take a very warm shower! Set your intention(s). Relax your muscles, feel the water, and allow the water to be a cleansing agent.
- Create! Paint, decorate, cook a new recipe—do something to inspire your creative juices.

It is up to you to decide what helps put your feet back on the ground. If you are unsure, pay attention to how you feel when you join in an activity. You can take some time to look through magazines and cut out what speaks to you. It could be a picture, fashion, a saying, or just a color. Put the pictures out before you on the floor and take the time to see what's close to your heart. That will be your "grounding list."

Essential oils are wonderful to get your feet back on the ground. Let's put together a blend of **clary sage, frankincense, lavender,** and **ylang ylang** and allow both their emotional and energetic properties to bring us back down.

FEET ON THE GROUND

2 tablespoons grape seed oil

2 drops clary sage (stimulates creativity; encourages focus)

3 drops frankincense (quiets the mind; promotes tranquility)

5 drops lavender (nurtures; balances all body systems)

1 drop ylang ylang (acts as a sedative and nervine)

Thoroughly blend all oils.

Apply 3–4 drops of the blend to the bottoms of both feet. Add 6–8 drops to unscented body lotion and massage all over your body after a shower or bath.

Put 1–2 drops of the blend in your hands, rub them together and cup your face to inhale slowly for a few minutes.

55. FRUSTRATION

We set goals to reach in our personal life or business careers and work hard to reach them. When we reach these goals we are elated. However, at times there are setbacks; some big, some small. The end result is frustration. We can let it motivate us to do better, but if we allow frustration to linger, it leads to anger, depression, lack of self-worth, lack of self-confidence, or defeatism.

Frustration is a part of life. If you can keep your goals small and attainable, then once you reach them, you can set larger ones. The important thing is not to allow frustration to control you. Learn to accept some situations, appreciate life's journey, and make necessary adjustments to your goals. Do this and you will possess a great secret that leads to happiness.

The support of essential oils will get you moving forward, bring balance, clear confusion, center the mind, build self-confidence, and keep you breathing! Let's look at **frankincense, lavender,** and **lemon**.

ACCEPTANCE

6 drops lavender (gets you moving forward; brings complete balance)

3 drops lemon (clears confusion; uplifts; makes way for positive emotional energy)

3 drops frankincense (encourages deep breathing; centers the mind)

Thoroughly blend all oils.

Massage 6–8 drops over your body. Then pour ½ cup of Epsom Salts directly under running water in the bathtub. When the tub is full, turn off the water and add 3 drops of the blend to the water. Soak in a warm bath for 20–30 minutes. Relax, accept, and be happy.

56. FRIGIDITY

Frigidity is sometimes referred to as Female Sexual Dysfunction. It is not an uncommon challenge to women at different times throughout their lives. It is more than lacking a sex drive; it can have emotional, physical, and/or medical origins and consequences.

Emotional distance from your partner may be due to unresolved feelings of past sexual assault, feelings of guilt or shame, boredom, or a lack of self image and confidence. Physical difficulties may result from discomfort during sexual intercourse, fatigue, hormone imbalance, or trauma from surgery. Medical origins of the condition may be from medications such as an antidepressant or birth control pills. The hormones of estrogen, progesterone, and testosterone decrease during menopause, which leads to a low libido.

Essential oils will add a much-needed warmth to help restore what has been lacking. **Clary sage, geranium, ginger,** and **ylang ylang** are four oils to consider. You can choose to make the following blend:

BEAUTIFUL WARMTH

2 tablespoons grape seed oil

3 drops clary sage (balances hormones; removes inhibitions)

3 drops geranium (balances hormones; encourages love of self, happiness)

3 drops ginger (a warming oil; increases libido)

1 drop ylang ylang (aphrodisiac; balances sexual emotion)

Thoroughly blend all oils. Locate a professional massage therapist in your area and take blend with you to be used. Human touch, without any sexual intent, is very important.

Add 2–3 drops to a warm bath.

Inhale the blend daily as your brain is your most important organ for sexual pleasure.

ESSENTIAL OILS TIP

If you are currently challenged with frigidity, do not hesitate to seek help from your partner, gynecologist, psychologist, or a professional therapist. If you are on medications, review the essential oils with your doctor and/or pharmacist for any contraindications.

57. GRIEF

No one is exempt from the pain of grief. Your tears will be bitter. The body needs to cleanse the toxic acids that build up within it. Don't resist tears, but allow their journey on your face to cover your stomach, lung, heart, and intestinal reflex and nerve points. Feel them and thank them.

If your grief is severe, there are a multitude of drugs and/or herbs to give you the support you will need. Seek professional medical or integrative help. Essential oils can also be your friends.

Your lungs and colon are affected by grief. If you become ill with a respiratory or digestive challenge know that your body is helping you by removing the negative emotions to make way for positive ones.

You can do a steam inhalation using 1 drop of eucalyptus oil in a bowl of hot water. Place a towel over your head and breathe in the aroma. This will clear the mucus and open your breathing passages.

Add 1 drop of eucalyptus and 1 drop of rosemary to 1 teaspoon of grape seed oil and rub on the bottoms of both your feet and over your chest. Do not use rosemary if you have epilepsy, a fever, are prone to seizures, or if you are pregnant and/or breastfeeding. You can substitute 1 drop of tea tree oil.

If you are experiencing anger, inhale lavender oil.

Draw a warm bath, turn off the water, add 3–4 drops of lavender, and soak for 15–20 minutes.

To help you work through feelings of depression, failure, or apathy add 2 drops of frankincense and 1 drop of geranium to 2 tablespoons of unscented face cream. Use this daily. You can also add the same amount of drops to a cotton ball and inhale when needed. Place the cotton ball in a zip lock bag to take with you during the day if needed.

58. GUILT

Knowingly or unknowingly, we will err in judgment and decisions, injuring others physically, mentally, emotionally, or spiritually. For the normal person with a conscience, the emotion that follows is guilt.

It takes courage and inner strength to make amends, but that will add beauty to your person. Unaddressed guilt eats away at your self-worth. Do not let that happen!

Once you have repaired the damage done, let it go. Allow the one you hurt to accept or deny your positive actions. It is no longer about you.

Geranium, lavender, and **lemon** can give you courage, inner strength, peace, and maintain your self-worth. Let's make a blend!

MAKING AMENDS

2 tablespoons grape seed oil

4 drops geranium (supports intimate communication; increases intuition)

6 drops lavender (reduces anxiety; nurturing; balances emotions)

2 drops lemon (uplifting and cleansing)

Thoroughly blend all oils.

Apply 4–6 drops over your body after a bath or shower. Make sure to massage over the chest area in a circular motion.

Inhale the blend while making plans to pursue peace.

59. DISAPPOINTMENT

An ancient proverb says, "Expectation postponed makes the heart sick." I have always thought of this as a perfect description of disappointment.

Disappointment may first manifest as anger. Sometimes you mask this with a false cheerfulness. Either way, if you linger in anger, you rob yourself of personal growth. This, in turn, will affect your health. Lungs, colon, heart, and small intestine will seek your attention. You may become sick with a respiratory illness, have inadequate bowel movements, or become lethargic. Instead, let your sadness make the journey needed. Set new goals and expectations. Do something new. Help another person.

The essential oils of **frankincense, lavender,** and **peppermint** will sustain you emotionally.

GENTLE RELEASE

2 tablespoons grape seed oil
4 drops frankincense (quiets the mind; focuses attention inward; stimulates tranquility)
6 drops lavender (calming; nurturing; soothing; balancing)
2 drops peppermint (uplifting; awakening; stimulates creativity and new ideas)

Thoroughly blend all oils.

Use 4–6 drops of the blend after a bath or shower.

Inhalation of the blend will bring immediate strength and confidence.

Massage 4–6 drops directly on the chest.

ESSENTIAL OILS TIP

There are times when disappointment leads to a deep depression. If that is the case with you, seek immediate professional help.

60. BETRAYAL

Betray, delude, or deceive. There are no pretty words to describe dishonest behavior. Betrayal by someone we love or a close friend can be emotionally numbing.

The following essential oils help work through the stages of rebuilding trust.

- **Clary sage** will move stagnant energy, calm the mind, help you make good decisions, and support emotional challenges.
- **Clove** is a beautiful warm oil for both body and mind as it restores self confidence. Do not use clove in a bath or if you have a blood clotting disorder.
- **Eucalyptus** is uplifting and cleansing for negative emotions. It aids in concentration and clearing the mind. Caution: This is a very potent oil that needs to be diluted in a carrier oil, 1 drop per 1 teaspoon.
- **Frankincense** quiets the mind and brings tranquility.
- **Geranium** will support intimate conversation and increase intuition.
- **Lavender** will reduce anxiety and fear, bringing back the balance needed.
- **Lemon** simultaneously uplifts and cleanses. Caution: If you use this oil in a skin preparation, be sure to cover up your skin when going outside as the oil will react to the sunlight, making your skin hypersensitive. Make sure your lemon oil is pure and not cloudy.
- **Peppermint** is awakening, uplifting, and promotes self-confidence.
- **Rosemary** will strengthen the mind and clear out negative thoughts to encourage clarity. Caution: If you have epilepsy, a fever, are prone to seizures, are pregnant and/or breastfeeding, do not use this oil.
- **Tea tree** builds strength, self-confidence, and uplifts the spirit. Caution: If your skin is sensitive, use 2 teaspoons of carrier oil and 2 drops of tea tree to dilute.
- **Ylang ylang** is an antidepressant, sedative, and nervine. This oil will assist you in regaining feelings of joy and pleasure. Caution: If you have low blood pressure, be cautious using this oil. Use a dilution of 1 drop per 1 teaspoon of carrier oil, as ylang ylang can be overpowering.

Choose up to three of the oils that best fit your emotional state. Make a small diluted blend using 2 tablespoons grape seed oil as your carrier. Add 1 drop of oil at a time until upon inhaling, it "speaks" to you. Apply on your chest and around the base of your neck and inhale deeply.

61. FEAR

Fear is a healthy response to life-threatening conditions. Your body will shut down systems that are not needed at that moment and release adrenalin, as well as send blood to your muscles. From youth to your maturing years, you face fear. The problem occurs when fear becomes paralyzing.

Essential oils can help you with everyday fears, traumatic fears, and overwhelming fears. Again, we will use oils that overlap with each other. We can use **clary sage, frankincense, geranium, lavender, lemon,** and **ylang ylang**.

QUIET BALANCE

2 tablespoons grape seed oil
2 drops frankincense (quiets the mind; encourages tranquility)
3 drops geranium (balances hormones)
6 drops lavender (soothing; reduces anxiety and fear; balances body systems)

Add 4–6 drops in a bath and soak for 15–20 minutes.

Put 2–3 drops on the bottoms of both feet before bed, or add 6–8 drops to your unscented body lotion and massage over your whole body.

ESSENTIAL OILS TIP

If you have experienced traumatic fear, add 2 drops of lemon and massage over the kidneys and bladder where the body deals with fear. It will also help eliminate excess adrenalin. If you feel very nervous or anxious, put 1 drop of ylang ylang on the bottoms of both feet for a sedative effect before lying down. Use only 1 drop per 1 teaspoon of carrier oil or body lotion.

62. CONFLICT

Some people enjoy conflict for its own sake. They have no insight, nor do they want any, as to how their actions affect others. When you work with or are in the presence of an argumentative person it is good to remember that it's not about you; it is all about them. If you're an argumentative person, recognize that conflict is something you use to protect yourself from getting too close to others.

Essential oils can bring an inner balance, clear away negative energy, and build healthy self-confidence. We will work with **geranium, frankincense, lavender, lemon,** and **ylang ylang**.

PURSUE PEACE

2 tablespoons grape seed oil

2 drops geranium (tonic for the nervous system)

2 drops frankincense (elevates your mood)

4 drops lavender (balances all systems; relaxing, nurturing)

2 drops lemon (clears away negative energy)

1 drop ylang ylang (builds self-confidence; supports inner equilibrium)

If you are in daily contact with an argumentative person, you can diffuse the recommended drops with the diffuser you are using. Also, place 3–4 drops of the blend onto a cotton ball and put in a plastic zip lock bag to take with you. Inhale as needed. When you return home, add 6–8 drops to unscented body lotion and massage over your body after a shower or bath.

If you are the argumentative person, make the cotton ball inhaler per previous instructions. Also, apply 3–4 drops of the blend to the bottoms of both feet at night before bed. After a bath or shower, massage 6–8 drops on the upper abdomen and deeply inhale.

63. MOURNING

Everyone has a story of a loved one who has died. For each individual person, the grief process is unique, but certain stages are common, similar to other forms of grief. These include anger, denial, emotional numbness, and depression. There is no one direction or order to these emotions. Life as you have known it has abruptly changed. There's no time limit for working through this loss; it's your own journey to be honored and respected.

You must take care of yourself no matter how hard that seems. Continue to eat, sleep, and exercise. Essential oils can have a tremendous affect on your mood, and your physical and mental health. Just inhaling them will bring instant comfort. The oils of **clary sage, frankincense, lavender,** and **peppermint** are a beginning. **Rose absolute–*Rosa damascena*** may prove to be a tonic for your heart. It will be an investment, but one worth making. You can massage 1–3 drops on your chest when grief overtakes you.

RESTORATIVE SPIRIT

2 tablespoons grape seed oil

4 drops clary sage (stimulates creativity; moves stagnant energy; supports emotional challenges)

4 drops frankincense (quiets the mind; brings focus; promotes tranquility)

6 drops lavender (calming, nurturing; reduces panic attacks; balances all body systems)

2 drops peppermint (uplifting and awakening; promotes self-confidence; clears stagnant energy)

Massage the blend over your whole body and especially the chest area. Use 3–5 drops and massage in a circular motion. Inhalation will be an important part of support, as well. Just place 2–5 drops of the blend on a cotton ball and deeply inhale when needed.

ESSENTIAL OILS TIP

If you are currently a caregiver or were a caregiver of a loved one, in addition to grief, you may be challenged with burnout. The information here does not replace medical or therapeutic counseling when needed. There is no shame in reaching out for such support.

64. NEGLECTED NERVOUS SYSTEM

Every system in our body is controlled by our nervous system. Yet, we sometimes fail to give thought or support to it. Look at your skin. Look under your eyes. Do you see lines in your face that weren't there last year? This is your body's nervous system forcing you to give it support.

Two of the best teas to drink for nerves are Stinging Nettle (or Nettle) and Oat Straw. These can be found at a reputable health food store. Combine them and drink them every day. You will notice a tranquil difference.

Applying a castor oil pack on your core, right below your breast area, once each week, will do wonders for your sleep, bowel movements, and attitude. In Section 3 you will find directions for making a castor oil pack.

Use **frankincense, lavender,** and **lemon**. They will prove to be nourishing, restorative, and uplifting to your nervous system.

NERVE SETTLER

2 tablespoons grape seed oil

3 drops frankincense (nervous system tonic; promotes nourishment and tranquility)

6 drops lavender (calming; balancing to all body systems; nurturing)

3 drops lemon (expands energy; uplifting, cleansing)

Thoroughly blend all oils.

Add 3 drops to your castor oil pack.

Add 3–6 drops to unscented body lotion and massage over your entire body.

Apply 2–5 drops to the bottom of each foot before bed.

Chapter 4
MENTAL AND SPIRITUAL WELLNESS

We were created with a need to worship. Some have faith in a Creator, a god, or other higher power they feel is worthy of their worship. Those who do not have a belief in such entities still worship someone or something. Whatever is the most important pursuit in their lives, money, material things, people, etc., this is their "god."

Humans have a need for a purpose in life and a compulsion to share that with others. How you go about this process to find out "Why am I here?" will be unique. Being true to yourself, being tolerant of other beliefs, and living according to your values and beliefs promote spiritual wellness. An openness to and deep appreciation of the world that surrounds you will deeply affect your spiritual health.

Mental wellness is both biological and social. We all have a family history of health challenges. Our nervous system, illness, and any medications we may be taking will affect our mental wellness. Socially, if we have been through great trauma, either physically, mentally, emotionally, or spiritually, our mental well-being is deeply affected. You can support your mental health by being physically active, getting proper rest, maintaining a healthy diet, controlling stress, and surrounding yourself with positive people and environments.

Essential oils can contribute to both areas of wellness. Spiritually, the oils ground us, support clear thinking, open our minds, help us focus when meditating, and displace negative influences. Mentally, they reduce mental fatigue, stimulate awareness, uplift, and nurture throughout emotional trauma.

65. STRESS

Not all stress is negative. If you are finding happiness in your job, helping others, being creative, raising your goals just a little bit higher, and this feels stimulating to your energy level, you are under stress . . . positive stress! No need to add support to that because it's all good.

However, when you become excessively tired, continuously irritable, start getting headaches, can't sleep, or experience pain, it's time to bring on the essential oils. Do not let these symptoms build until you collapse.

You can use the essential oils of **geranium, lavender,** and **lemon** to banish depression, increase imagination, reduce anxiety, instill a balance within the body, and bring "happy" back.

Add 3–5 drops of the blend to unscented body lotion and liberally apply after a bath or shower.

Place 3–5 drops of the blend on a cotton ball, put in plastic zip lock bag to take with you and inhale as needed. Especially good if you are about to take a test or complete work on an intricate project.

If your teenage child is involved with after-school activities, the following blend can help with the stress they undergo but may not want to talk about. It will also be beneficial for balancing their ever-changing hormones. It's named for a very special teenager who assisted me with this blend.

MESS WITH STRESS

2 tablespoons grape seed oil

7 drops geranium (anti-depressant, increases imagination; opens up the sensory world)

7 drops lavender (anti-depressant; reduces anxiety, calms, nurtures; balances all body systems)

4 drops lemon (the "happy" oil, uplifts, cleanses; expands energy outward)

Thoroughly blend all the oils. Inhale, inhale, inhale!

THE KENNY G EFFECT

2 tablespoons grape seed oil

3 drops clary sage

5 drops lemon

3 drops frankincense

Thoroughly blend all oils.

Massage 4–6 drops of the blend all over your body after a shower or bath.

Place 3–4 drops of the blend on a cotton ball, put in a zip lock bag, and take with you to inhale when needed.

66. EMOTIONAL TRAUMA

Today there is no shortage of divorce, illness, natural disasters, domestic abuse, abandonment, and death. All of these and more take a heavy toll on our emotions and mental state. It may take a long time for such wounds to heal, and they may show up in lack of sleep, lack of trust, anger, depression, low self-esteem, and oversensitivity. The oils chosen from this book will help therapeutically, emotionally, and energetically to sidestep these negative effects.

BE SET FREE

2 tablespoons grape seed oil

3 drops geranium (antidepressant; opens the sensory world; supports intimate communication)

5 drops lavender (antidepressant; nurturing; reduces anxiety and fear; balances all body systems)

2 drops peppermint (uplifting and awakening; supports self-confidence and creativity; clears negative energy)

1 drop ylang ylang (antidepressant; sedative and nervine for emotional shock)

Thoroughly blend all oils.

Apply 2–3 drops of the blend to the bottoms of both feet before bed.

After a shower or bath, massage 6–8 drops over your entire body, concentrating over the chest area.

Place 2–4 drops of blend on a cotton ball and inhale as needed.

ESSENTIAL OILS TIP

Store peppermint away from any homeopathic remedies as it may dull their effectiveness. Always keep the dilution low for peppermint. If you are prone to low blood pressure, feel free to replace the ylang ylang with 2 drops of clary sage. Always seek medical and/or integrative professional help if your symptoms increase, interfere with your daily activities, or become life threatening.

67. THE BLAHS

Have you ever felt as if you just wanted to stay in bed, not see anyone or do anything? Everyone experiences this at least once in their lives. It's okay. Having the "blahhhhuesss" can be positive . . . for a couple of days. Then, you just have to force yourself out of that bed. Do some stretching or gentle exercise and you will begin to feel better. After an uplifting shower, cook yourself something. And, last but not least, laugh. Your diaphragm has missed you!

What essential oils can we concoct to use in our shower to lift our energy, get our creative juices flowing, put a smile on our face, all the while being grounded? How about **clary sage, frankincense, lemon,** and **peppermint**?

BLUES AWAY

2 tablespoons grape seed oil

4 drops clary sage (stimulates creativity)

2 drops frankincense (helps you be contentedly grounded)

2 drops lemon (brings on the smile)

2 drops peppermint (the wake-up ingredient)

Thoroughly blend all oils.

After a shower, put 4–6 drops in your hands, cup your face and inhale deeply 3–4 times. Then, massage all over your body, especially around the temple area and the back of your neck. Let the day begin!

ESSENTIAL OILS TIP

Store peppermint away from all homeopathic remedies as it may weaken their effect.

68. MENTAL FATIGUE

Do you recall driving in fog so thick you had to struggle and strain to see immediately in front of you? It happens in our heads sometimes. Brain fog! We get confused, can't focus or remember, and thinking just hurts.

The reasons for this vary. If you find that this is becoming chronic and interfering with your professional and personal life, secure the appropriate medical and/or integrative help. In this chapter, we will work with sleep, hormonal balance, and stress.

It's amazing that when we allow our bodies the restorative sleep needed, we wake up feeling so good and yet our body has worked all night! Menopause plays with our hormones so if we can support a healthy balance using essential oils, our hormones will play nice. We can control our reactions to stress so that everyday happenings will not tear at our inner or outer self.

We can keep our oils simple and concise. Using **geranium, rosemary,** and **peppermint** we can lift the fog.

FOG FREE

2 tablespoons grape seed oil

4 drops geranium (balances hormones; stimulates creativity; supports energetic mental challenges)

2 drops peppermint (uplifting and awakening; clears stagnant energy)

4 drops rosemary (stimulates memory; energizing and uplifting)

Thoroughly blend all oils.

After putting 2–4 drops in your hands, cup your face and inhale deeply a couple of times. Massage over your entire body after a shower or bath.

Add 3–4 drops of the blend to warm bath water once the water is turned off. Relax in the bath 15–30 minutes.

Place 2–3 drops on a cotton ball, put in a zip lock plastic bag to take with you, and inhale when needed.

ESSENTIAL OILS TIP

Store peppermint away from homeopathic remedies as it may weaken their effectiveness. If you have epilepsy, a fever, are prone to seizures, or are pregnant and/or breastfeeding, do not use rosemary. Replace it with 4 drops of lavender.

69. MENTAL ACCURACY

If you can focus, memorize, concentrate, and comprehend what you see and read you have mental accuracy, or mental acuity. Various parts of the brain must be active for us to have and maintain mental acuity.

Do a crossword puzzle. No matter your age, continue to learn new things. If you have wanted to learn a musical instrument or take an art class, do it. When you feel a little disorganized inside yourself, look around at your environment. Is there clutter in your bedroom, closet, office, kitchen, or living area? Where there is clutter outside, there will be clutter inside you. Take 15–20 minutes a day and become clutter free. This is a most "freeing" thing to do for yourself. Also, by making lists and keeping your important items in the same place you can maintain your mental acuity.

Essential oils offer very good support. The best way to use them is to inhale them. So choose 1–2 that resonate with you from the following list, and make a cotton ball inhaler by adding a combined total of 2–3 drops of your oil(s). Or, add a combined total of 3–5 drops of oil(s) in an unscented body lotion before applying it on your body. You can use these daily to allow them to be a healthy mental maintenance.

- **Frankincense**—quiets the mind, bringing focused attention and tranquility.
- **Lavender**—reduces anxiety; calming, soothing and total body balancing.
- **Lemon**—simultaneously uplifts and cleanses.
- **Peppermint**—stimulates creativity, new ideas and self-confidence. Caution: Store separate from homeopathic remedies as it may dull their effectiveness.
- **Rosemary**—strengthens the mind; clears negative thoughts and encourages clarity. Caution: If you have epilepsy, a fever, are prone to seizures, or are pregnant and/or breastfeeding, do not use this oil.

70. MEDITATION

Meditation and spiritual wellness go hand in hand. With meditation our body eliminates stress and at the same time prevents more stress from entering the body! We decrease anxiety, become focused, and solve problems, and this leads to being emotionally happy.

Spiritually, meditation can strengthen our relationship with our Creator and bring inner peace. To benefit the most, allow meditation to be a part of every day, even just 10–15 minutes; you will not only look forward to that time, but you will grow spiritually.

The essential oils of **clary sage, lavender,** and **frankincense** can be blended equally together as follows:

INTENTIONAL LINGERING

4 drops clary sage (calms the mind; moves stagnant energy)

4 drops frankincense (quiets the mind; focuses attention; supports tranquility)

4 drops lavender (calming and balancing)

Thoroughly blend all oils. Place 4 drops of the blend in a diffuser of your choice and keep it close by. Or, if you do not have a diffuser, add 4 drops of the blend to a bowl of hot water.

71. PERSONAL GROWTH

Personal growth is, well, personal. It is all about you. What makes you happy? What goals do you have? What are your strengths and weaknesses? Where is your heart? What is your priority in life? What is your favorite food? Who do you love the most? What motivates you?

How do you keep personally growing? One way is to truthfully answer the preceding questions. If you do not have the answers to all or even to some, take the time to explore for yourself. Maintain a balance in your life with both strengths and weaknesses. Both are needed for personal growth.

The essential oils of **clary sage, clove, lemon,** and **ylang ylang** can support you with self-confidence, positive energy, creativity, and inner depth.

PRIVATE EXPANSION

2 tablespoons grape seed oil

4 drops clary sage (stimulates creativity; assists with indecisiveness; calming)

1 drop clove (warms both mind and body; builds self-confidence)

2 drops lemon (uplifting, cleansing)

1 drop ylang ylang (assists with feelings of joy—a "heart" oil; sedative)

Thoroughly blend all oils.

Add 2–3 drops to a warm bath after the water is turned off. Soak for 15–20 minutes. After a shower or bath, apply 6–8 drops to your hands, cup your face, inhale, and then massage over your entire body.

ESSENTIAL OILS TIP

If you have a blood clotting disorder or are on a medical regimen, do not use clove oil. You can substitute 3 drops of lavender oil.

72. PROTECTION FROM NEGATIVE INFLUENCES

Negativity isn't always packaged as loud, aggressive, pushy, or overbearing. Sometimes it's shy, charming, or even alluring. Whatever the form, it leaves us spiritually and mentally drained. A negative person will complain, be dramatic with the smallest things, blame others, and hurtfully gossip about someone you mutually know.

The best way to protect yourself is to limit the time you spend in their company. That means setting boundaries and keeping them. If you do not wish to discuss a topic brought up, honestly let them know you do not wish to be a part of the discussion. If you remain calm, they will calm down. Don't try to fix them; that's their job.

The essential oils to help you have self-worth, courage, and mental strength are **frankincense, ginger, lavender, peppermint,** and **rosemary**. Once you decide which oil is your "go to" oil for combating negativity, place 2–4 drops of your oil on a cotton ball and inhale. If you know you will be meeting up with a negative person, take the cotton ball with you in a zip lock bag and inhale before, during, and after contact with them. You may even notice the person becoming more positive as you take care of yourself and they inhale it inadvertently, too!

Do not use rosemary if you have epilepsy, are prone to seizures, are pregnant, and/or breastfeeding.

73. AWARENESS

Do you talk to yourself? It can be a great learning experience, especially when dealing with "triggers" in your life. If you lack self-awareness, you allow your emotions to dictate your reaction rather than using your reason to digest, grow, and become stronger.

How can you develop self-awareness? First breathe deeply and in minutes you'll become calmer. Ask yourself, "What am I feeling, and where is it centered?" Remember that you are safe. Then, become the observer. You will develop empathy for yourself. This empathy will then allow you to control the emotion instead of the emotion controlling you.

The essential oils to give you strength of mind and awareness, self-confidence and courage are:

- **Clary sage** (moves stagnant energy; calms nervous anxiety; supports emotional challenges)
- **Eucalyptus** (uplifting; cleanses negative emotions and energy)
- **Frankincense** (quiets the mind; brings focus and tranquility)
- **Lavender** (calming and nurturing; reduces anxiety and fear; balances all body systems)
- **Peppermint** (uplifting, awakening; supports self-confidence)
- **Tea tree** (builds strength, self-confidence and uplifts the spirit)

Choose the oil(s) best suited for your end goal.

Eucalyptus and Peppermint are good for inhalation.

Add 3 drops of frankincense, 3 drops of lavender, and 2 drops of tea tree to 2 tablespoons of your body cream and massage over your body after a bath or shower. If you find you are more sensitive or more "triggers" are occurring, use the massage cream daily and choose a blend for inhaling when needed.

74. MENTAL GROWTH

It is healthy to expand your mental and spiritual wellness throughout your life. This is a never-ending project.

If you take good care of your body, it will take good care of you. So eating nutritious food, performing new exercises, hydrating yourself, and getting restorative sleep are essential. It has been said that laughter is the best medicine as it improves your immune system and relaxes the body. Prayer is also a wonderful gift for relaxation and for reducing stress. Always keep your goals small and attainable to have a good foundation to build upon. Never shy away from seeking help when you need it.

For essential oils, the combination of **clary sage, lavender,** and **lemon** may be just the "lift" you need.

EXPANSION

2 tablespoons grape seed oil

3 drops clary sage (moves stagnant energy; stimulates creativity; calming and supportive emotionally)

4 drops lavender (nurturing, balancing; reduces anxiety and stress)

3 drops lemon (full of outward, expanding energy)

Thoroughly blend all oils.

Daily after a shower or bath, add 3–5 drops to unscented body lotion and massage your body. Or take the blend with you for a professional massage. Apply 3–5 drops on the bottoms of both feet at night before bed.

ESSENTIAL OILS TIP

Lemon will react to sunlight and may cause burning or skin damage. Therefore, if you use this blend before going outside during the day, just make sure to cover up for a couple hours. Also, always use lemon oil that is fresh and not cloudy.

75. OPEN MIND

To be open-minded doesn't mean accepting everything others say and do. There is good and bad, right and wrong, and taking a stand for what you believe is important. However, you can still be open-minded and not dogmatic. Everyone has the gift of free will. To be open-minded you need to find common ground with the other person, as big or little as that common ground may be.

No one person knows everything, and we can learn from each other. Having an open mind will allow internal growth, and you will look for ways to show kindness to others. To have an appreciation of others' likes, dislikes, backgrounds, and culture will richly increase your own strength.

The essential oil for open mindedness is **lavender**. Lavender is nurturing, soothing and brings balance to all body systems, yet it will stay true to its therapeutic properties, emotionally and energetically.

You can use lavender in your bath by adding 2–3 drops to the water after you turn off the faucet.

Place 2–3 drops on a cotton ball for a quick and easy inhaler.

Apply 2–3 drops "neat" on the bottom of each foot before bed.

Add 3–5 drops to an unscented body lotion for all-over body massage.

PART 3

BEAUTY

Chapter 5
SKINCARE AND HAIRCARE

Skin is one of the busiest organs the body has. It provides protection from outside dangers, is our heating and cooling system, and provides stimuli to the brain through nerve endings. If there is an internal imbalance, it will generally show up on our skin.

Huge amounts of money are spent on very expensive skin treatments, but let's save our money and use essential oils. They will ward off infection, improve circulation, and even oxygenate the skin. Essential oils will bring needed nourishment on a cellular level to the skin. By using essential oils instead of manmade chemicals, you'll make a dramatic difference and will feel so good.

Remember: If you nourish the inside, your outside will flourish in every way. This is such a fun part of the book. Let's play!

76. ACNE

As we reach puberty our body goes through numerous hormonal changes. One of these affects the overproduction of fat from the sebaceous glands and produces the skin condition called acne. Acne is not just for the young; many continue to be challenged with it throughout their lives, especially during menstruation. It not only shows up on the face, but can affect arms, back, neck, and chest. It is painful and sometimes will leave deep scars behind.

It begins with a blackhead that turns into a pimple with lots of "oozy gooey" stuff inside. The temptation to pop the pimple and squeeze out the interior is great. However, when we do this, chances are we're infecting the skin around the pimple, nurturing new acne. Eating a clean diet of fruits and vegetables and eliminating caffeine, alcohol, and (I'm sorry!) chocolate, especially at times of flare up, will go a long way toward controlling your acne.

Let's blend some essential oils from this book to jazz things up. We will use **clary sage, lavender,** and **tea tree**.

JAZZY GIRL

2 tablespoons jojoba oil

3 drops clary sage (antiseptic, sebum regulating)

5 drops lavender (stimulates growth of new cells; antibacterial, antiviral; prevents scarring; analgesic—numbs pain)

2 drops tea tree (antiseptic, anti-infectious, antifungal)

Thoroughly blend all oils together.

Cleanse the face with a pure, nonchemical product. Then very gently apply the blend over the affected area on the face, neck, back, arms, or chest. Do this in the morning and in the evening.

ESSENTIAL OILS TIP

We will be using jojoba oil (wax)–*Simmondsia chinensis* as the carrier oil for all blends for the skin. Jojoba is a natural sebum (almost identical to our skin's natural oil). It is odorless, an antioxidant, will not go rancid, and supports the shelf life of the essential oils used in the blend. Purchase organic jojoba from a reputable aromatherapy business.

77. DRY SKIN

Leather. That is what dry skin looks like. Tight. That is what dry skin feels like. Why does our skin become so dry? Hormonal imbalance, the sebaceous glands not producing enough fatty oil, and stress. Without the fluid of the needed fat, the skin becomes lifeless and begins to flake off. Staying hydrated is very important, so along with drinking water, add fruits to your diet that are high in liquid content such as watermelon, cucumbers, and berries (if it's wintertime, add frozen berries to a smoothie). Contact a local skincare specialist to help you add the right amount of omega-3 and vitamin B.

We will use the essential oils of **geranium, lavender,** and **lemon** to bring needed nourishment to dry skin.

HYDRATE THY SKIN

2 tablespoons jojoba oil

4 drops geranium (regulates oil production; improves skin elasticity)

5 drops lavender (regenerates new skin cells; nourishes dry skin)

2 drops lemon (soothing to dry skin; supports healthy skin)

Thoroughly blend all the oils together.

After cleansing the skin, apply the blend to your skin in gentle strokes. If after a couple of minutes there remains a bit of oil, gently wipe off. Use this both in the morning and evening. Remember that lemon is photosensitizing, so when going outside, make sure to stay covered for a couple hours.

ESSENTIAL OILS TIP

Commercial soap is very drying to the skin. You can easily make your own oil-based cleanser by putting together equal parts of organic olive oil, organic castor oil, and organic grape seed oil. Feel free to add 2–3 drops of an essential oil for your skin. This will not clog pores and will leave your skin feeling nourished.

78. OILY SKIN

Our overactive sebaceous glands are adding to the excess oil on our skin. Hormones are unbalanced, puberty has set in, and our skin is shiny. Of course, you don't need to be pubescent to experience oily skin; puberty just happens to be the beginning of great hormonal changes affecting the skin. When our skin gets oily we wash it again and again. Over-the-counter products may contain alcohol and many harsh chemicals. These creams may temporarily decrease the oil but will have bad side effects. So, let's make a very easy organic cleanser for your skin using organic raw honey and lemon essential oil.

HONEY AND LEMON CLEANSER

2 tablespoons raw organic honey (balances pH; hydrates)
8 drops lemon (antibacterial; astringent)

Gently warm the honey in a double boiler until it is a smooth, relatively thin liquid. Let it cool for a couple minutes before adding the lemon oil. Thoroughly blend the oil and honey. Store in an air tight container.

Place a small amount (the size of a nickel) on closed finger tips, add 3–4 drops of water on top of blend, and the stickiness will immediately be gone.

Gently apply over face and let it penetrate skin for a few minutes. Take a shower and before getting out, gently wipe the cleanser off your face. Then, apply a small amount of the following blend to cleansed skin:

2 tablespoons jojoba oil
3 drops tea tree (antibacterial; regulates oil production)
1 drop ylang ylang (regulates oil production; regenerates skin cells)

Thoroughly blend all oils. Apply a small amount to your face. If you get too much of the blend on your face, gently wipe it off.

You can use this both in the morning and evening.

79. COMBINATION SKIN

If you have an area on your face that is oily around the "T" zone (nose and forehead), more than likely you have combination skin. Due to the excess oil around the nose, you may see small blackheads forming, so give that area a little more TLC by using a gentle scrub. A great treat for combination skin is a facial steam. You can purchase a professional facial steamer online or be creative at home with 1–2 quarts boiling water in a heatproof, nonslip bowl. Sit comfortably with your hair pulled off your face, bend near the bowl, and drape a large towel over your head, keeping your eyes closed. Relax for 10–15 minutes, letting the steam and oils do their work. Do not put your face directly over the steam; you will need to adjust the distance based on your comfort level. When finished, use a cool splash of water or soft moist cloth to clean your face. Follow this with your favorite essential oil blend for your skin.

STEAM CLEANSING

2 tablespoons jojoba oil

4 drops clary sage (improves skin elasticity; tightens skin; promotes blood circulation)

3 drops lavender (regenerates skin cells; lightens age spots)

2 drops ylang ylang (helps regenerate skin cells; smoothing the appearance of fine lines; improves skins elasticity)

Thoroughly blend all oils. Only use *one* teaspoon of the blend for each facial steam you do. You can keep the remaining blend in a dark glass container with a tight-fitting lid. You will be able to do 6 facial steams with this blend.

80. SENSITIVE SKIN

Allergies to food, environment, products, or pets can irritate sensitive skin. Anyone who suffers from this will know almost immediately if she is in the wrong place or has just applied the wrong product. Your skin will turn red and may swell a bit, and you may even get a rash after you cleanse your face. The change in seasons may be beautiful to watch and enjoy, but can wreak havoc on our skin. Spring and summer are full of sunny days that may burn the skin. Fall and winter bring dry, cold air and wind that can dry out our skin, along with dry indoor heating, making it sensitive.

A mask of honey and yogurt may become your best friend through all the seasons. You can use ¼ cup of raw organic honey and 2 tablespoons of nonflavored, organic Greek yogurt (make sure it has all the fat). Blend them together into a smooth paste and apply to your face and neck. You can lie down and rest for 15–20 minutes, or if you need to get something done, feel free to go about your business. If any happens to get in your mouth, enjoy! The mask will become dry, so use warm water and a soft cloth to gently remove it. Your skin will be so happy. Then, thoroughly blend the following oils and apply over your face and neck for added nurturing:

2 tablespoons jojoba oil
4 drops geranium (improves skin elasticity; tightens skin; promotes blood circulation)
6 drops lavender (regenerates skin cells; balances all skin types)

81. ANTI-WRINKLE

Usually, sooner than later our wrinkles take us by surprise. There are wrinkles from a good, happy life and wrinkles that will appear from neglecting our health and wellbeing. So, how can we be proactive and give attention to our wrinkles?

Pay attention to what you choose to put into your body. What goes in must come out and not always in the way you think. Smoking, excess alcohol, junk food, depression, and stress will all claim a spot on your face and body.

Here are the integrative anti-wrinkle winners: **clary sage, frankincense, geranium, lavender,** and **lemon**. Let's make a blend.

INTEGRATIVE SKIN ANTI-AGING POTION

2 tablespoons jojoba oil

2 drops clary sage (improves skin elasticity; tightens skin; promotes blood circulation)

2 drops frankincense (natural toner; protects existing cells; encourages new cell growth; reduces the appearance of wrinkles; tightens skin)

3 drops geranium (improves skin elasticity; reduces appearance of wrinkles; promotes blood circulation to the application area)

5 drops lavender (regenerates skin cells; balances all skin types)

1 drop lemon (antibacterial, astringent)

Thoroughly blend all oils together.

Use before going to bed and apply over the face, neck, and shoulders. If you have wrinkles appearing on other parts of your body, apply some of the blend directly on them.

ESSENTIAL OILS TIP

Once you reach your Fabulous Forties and beyond, a lovely carrier oil to add to your blend is evening primrose oil—*Oenothera biennis*. This is a natural antioxidant and will keep other oils from turning rancid. Feel free to add this oil to any body cream you are using to bring rejuvenation to the skin. Always keep this oil tightly sealed, and in a cool, dark, dry area. Another carrier oil worth checking out at this time and beyond is carrot seed oil—*Daucus carota var. sativa*. It is a fixed oil, cold pressed from the seeds. This is a good oil for all skin types—it is absorbed quickly, and helps with wrinkles and so much more. If you store this oil in a cool, dry place it should last you for two years! Caution: Do not confuse this with the essential oil carrot seed–*Daucus carota*—because the process in obtaining the oil differs and thus the therapeutic properties also differ. Always pay attention to the Latin names for oils to be sure you purchase the correct one.

82. LIP CARE

Lips are so impressive. You can kiss all you want, make funny faces, and smile and they never wear out! They are fascinating except when they are cracked, or have a sore on them, or there are lines all around. Because the skin on our lips is very thin, we need to give it some additional support to keep it happy, healthy, and working. The most common challenge is chapped lips. Coming in second—cold sores. For dry, cracked lips we can use geranium and lavender. For any cold sores that appear we can use lemon and tea tree.

KISSABLE LIPS

1 ounce of white beeswax or organic shea butter

10 drops jojoba oil

5 drops geranium (anti-inflammatory and cooling; antibacterial, antiseptic)

5 drops lavender (antiseptic, analgesic— numbs pain; heals open wounds; stops bleeding)

Melt beeswax or shea butter in the microwave, approximately 30–60 seconds. Remove and add jojoba oil. Stir together. As it cools down, add the geranium and lavender. Fill a tin or small plastic container with the blend, refrigerate if you want it to harden quicker. Then, just use as needed.

You can use this on a daily basis for lovely lips.

If you have a cold sore, make the same blend, omit the geranium and lavender, and use 5 drops each of lemon and tea tree. Put directly on the sores. If you want to use the tea tree "neat" (without diluting) you can try that first. Just add a drop on the end of a cotton swab and apply directly on the sore(s).

ESSENTIAL OILS TIP

For a temporary lip "plumper" rub a dry washcloth over your lips to bring the blood to the surface. Don't rub too hard; just gently encourage the circulation of blood into your lips. Then add one to two drops of cinnamon leaf–*Cinnamomum selenium* to your Kissable Lips Blend and apply. Do not ingest cinnamon leaf oil. There may be a temporary burning sensation but it will stop. If the burning sensation does not stop, then wipe off.

83. REDUCING SKIN PIGMENTATION

Overexposure to sun, allergies, aging, heredity, medications, and sometimes skin cancer are common causes of skin pigmentation, or abnormal skin colorations. If you have a suspicious discoloration or spot on your skin, see a dermatologist immediately to rule out anything serious.

We'll work with two oils: **lavender** and **lemon**. Lavender is antiseptic and antifungal and effectively manages burns, acne, and blemishes. Lemon also is antiseptic and antibacterial, as well as an astringent, and rejuvenates dull skin. Using lemon on a regular basis will lighten and brighten the complexion while simultaneously adding protection to the skin from an assortment of challenges. Lemon will need to be diluted, as it is acidic, but that is also what makes it an almost instant skin brightener.

LIGHTENING BLEND

¼ cup of jojoba oil
4 drops lavender
3 drops lemon

Thoroughly blend all oils together.

Apply directly on the areas of pigmentation and leave on for 30–40 minutes. Then, cleanse skin and apply a skin moisturizer. Repeat once a day until you start to see results. Then, do a weekly maintenance treatment for your skin pigmentation. Use a sunscreen or cover-up to prevent additional pigmentation.

84. NEGLECTED FEET

We take our precious feet for granted by thinking they just support our body. However, feet have a huge impact on our overall health. Our circulatory system flows down to our feet and is pushed back up through use of our leg and pelvic muscles to reach the brain and heart. When we wear ill-fitting shoes, walk on concrete, or ignore internal body pains, the circulatory system slows down as crystals form in the feet. There are times when we think our feet hurt, but in reality they're getting our attention to support another system in the body. For example, if you have pain in the arch area of your foot, ask yourself if you are currently constipated. There is also evidence that bunions, calluses, corns, ingrown toenails, and the shape of our toes have a bearing on our emotional health.

So, we can make a relaxing foot soak and follow this with a massage oil using **geranium, peppermint,** and **lavender**.

HEALTHY FOOT SOAK

2 tablespoons Epsom Salts
3 drops geranium (anti-inflammatory, antispasmodic; supports urinary and liver detoxing)

3 drops peppermint (analgesic— numbs pain; anti-inflammatory, cooling; strengthens the liver and digestive systems)
3 drops lavender (analgesic, antibacterial, anti-inflammatory; soothing)

Fill a footbath with very warm, but not hot, water. Add the Epsom Salts and let them dissolve. Once dissolved, add the geranium, peppermint, and lavender. Soak your feet 10–15 minutes. After drying feet off, massage them with the following blend:

HEALTHY FOOT MASSAGE

2 tablespoons jojoba oil
6 drops geranium
8 drops lavender
6 drops peppermint

Thoroughly blend all oils. Massage on both feet after soaking.

ESSENTIAL OILS TIP

Store peppermint oil separately from homeopathic remedies as it may diminish their properties.

85. ITCHY SKIN

Few things drive us crazier than itchy skin. The more you scratch it, the more it itches. You could be dealing with an allergic reaction to food, an insect bite, contact with a poisonous plant, or dry skin. If you scratch your skin long enough, you'll break it, leaving you open to bacteria and infections.

When your skin is this itchy, you need to provide immediate comfort and support. A base blend of jojoba and castor oil can supply the intense moisturizing needed, and it is antibacterial, anti-fungal, and will assist in restoring healthy skin. **Eucalyptus, lavender,** and **peppermint** can then be added as follows:

SKIN ITCH BE GONE

1 tablespoon jojoba oil

1 tablespoon castor oil

2 drops eucalyptus (analgesic—numbs pain; antibacterial, antiviral)

8 drops lavender (antibacterial, antiseptic, analgesic; stops bleeding, cleans wounds, nurtures skin)

2 drops peppermint (analgesic, anti-inflammatory, antiseptic; cooling)

Thoroughly blend all oils.

Massage directly onto itchy skin. Repeat as needed until itchiness dissipates and/or open wounds are healed.

ESSENTIAL OILS TIP

Eucalyptus is a powerful essential oil. Do not use more drops than indicated. Peppermint oil may nullify the effects of homeopathic remedies, so keep it stored separately.

86. UNDER-EYE CONDITIONING

Our eyes are the windows to our souls. To keep them inviting takes care. You can spend hundreds of dollars on them and still live with bags, crow's feet, dark circles, and dryness.

When you use any product around your eyes you should use your ring finger with the least amount of pressure. The skin will respond well to a gentle, smooth touch. The same holds true when you cleanse your face. Be gentle and soft around your eyes.

A simple synergy blend to make for around the eyes appropriate for any age group consists of **jojoba oil, lavender, lemon,** and **vitamin E**. You can purchase vitamin E in capsule form and prick it open with a sterile needle or pin, allowing the oil to pour into your blend. Here's the recipe:

ALL ABOUT THE EYES

2 tablespoons jojoba oil

4 drops lavender (regenerates skin cells; anti-inflammatory; cooling, balancing)

2 drops lemon (antibacterial, astringent; brightens skin, regenerates skin cells)

1 capsule vitamin E (antioxidant; restores collagen, repairs skin cells)

Thoroughly blend all oils.

Using your ring finger, gently apply the blend around the eyes (not on eyelid). Do not get the oils into the eyes. Leave on for a few minutes, then wipe off excess. Any excess oil, even if it is the most wonderful oil, will pull down on the skin, so be sure to gently wipe off any excess oil. This recipe should allow for 8 treatments, so you can store the remaining blend in a dark glass container with a lid that seals tight. If you happen to do a weekly mask treatment, add this to the treatment.

ESSENTIAL OILS TIP

If you have puffy eyes or dark shadows, make a cup of green tea and allow it to cool in the refrigerator. Once cold, use cotton balls to dab around the eyes. Or, if you have the time, soak cotton make up remover pads in the tea, squeeze out the excess, and place on top of closed eyes for 10–15 minutes.

87. CELLULITE

Cellulite is connected to the hormone estrogen. This is a protective hormone that carries toxins and waste away from vital organs, especially reproductive organs. When it doesn't know what to do with a toxin, the estrogen will deposit it far away from the reproductive system—in hips, thighs, buttocks . . . are you seeing the picture? Men do not get cellulite because they do not produce estrogen.

Think about all the toxins we have in our food, air, and water. Some we can prevent; others we cannot. You can make positive changes that will encourage your body to begin releasing cellulite. Clean up your diet with fresh organic fruits and vegetables. Drink lots of water. **Dry brush** your skin daily. Keep in mind that you didn't get cellulite overnight, so getting rid of it will take time. There is a good oil blend to make from our list in this book.

epilepsy, are prone to seizures, are pregnant, and/or breastfeeding, do not use rosemary. Substitute with 3 drops juniper–Juniperus communis. Be sure to purchase juniper with this Latin name so as not to confuse it with other species.

Thoroughly blend all oils.

After you dry brush, shower, and when you get out of the shower, massage the blend using small circular motions on all areas of the body that have cellulite dimples. Allow the oils to penetrate the skin. Do not wipe off. If you are consistent with this protocol, you will see results very soon. Do not give up. Remember, if you begin this protocol and the cellulite starts to look even worse (because it's moving through the body's lymphatic system), celebrate because it's working. Just hang in there.

DIMPLES AWAY

2 tablespoons jojoba or grape seed oil

6 drops geranium (skin toner; improves blood circulation; detoxifies body systems; balances hormones)

3 drops rosemary (diuretic; stimulates circulation; encourages lymphatic system to drain away toxins) Caution: If you have

88. TICK REPELLENT

Ticks are not to be taken lightly. Once they begin sucking blood from humans or animals they may leave behind extremely dangerous unwanted guests in the body. If you remove a tick and a red ring appears around the bite, this is called a "bull's-eye" tick rash. Immediately visit your doctor and get the necessary antibiotics. If you have an integrative health practitioner, she or he can supplement the antibiotics with natural herbs. The seriousness of a tick bite cannot be overstated. Once you remove a tick you can apply lavender "neat" (no carrier needed) directly onto the bite. Repeat this once every 10 minutes for about an hour. This will begin warding off infection, pain, and swelling.

You can also make a great nontoxic tick repellent spray:

TICK'D OFF

½ ounce vodka

1½ ounce of distilled water

1 tablespoon vegetable glycerin

10 drops eucalyptus

12 drops lavender

10 drops lemon

10 drops peppermint

In a 2-ounce plastic (PET) spray bottle add vodka and essential oils. Shake together. Then add the vegetable glycerin and distilled water. Shake again. Store in the refrigerator and before using, shake the bottle and spray over your entire body.

ESSENTIAL OILS TIP

If you want to make this spray effective against mosquitoes, too, just add 8 drops of citronella–*Cymbopogon nardus* to the recipe. Do not be surprised if you notice that you feel wonderful, as all of these oils have beautiful emotional and energetic qualities. Citronella is also very useful against head lice.

89. ANT REPELLENT

Spring has sprung and summer is knocking on the door! Everything is coming to life and getting active again, including ants. It's incredible how they find their way into our homes. If we do nothing to repel them, they multiply by the thousands overnight. But, never fear, essential oils are here.

In a 2-ounce plastic (PET) spray bottle add the following in order:

ANTS AWAY

16 drops lavender

14 drops peppermint

½ ounce vodka

1½ ounces distilled water

Shake well and spray in the corners, cupboards, or cracks on floor where the ants are entering. Store in the refrigerator and use as needed.

ESSENTIAL OILS TIP

If you want to just use a single oil "neat" in an area, choose peppermint. Just put a couple of drops onto the area of entrance! Works immediately.

90. SUNBURN REMEDY

A healthy glow looks good unless it's really, really red! At this point it will be indicative of damage done to the skin, not to mention there will be a lot of pain. If you are burned that deeply you will need immediate medical intervention. For milder cases of sunburn, you can use essential oils.

Sit in a bathtub of cold water for about 10–15 minutes. Fluids are absolutely necessary, so drink lots of water. You may want to alternate water with fluids containing electrolytes if you have become dehydrated. Once out of the cold bath, apply **lavender** "neat" directly on the burn. One drop will go far, so use good common sense and thoroughly cover the burned area. Your skin will need to be nourished, so make the following blend to use over the next couple of days:

SKIN, "SO SORRY"

2 tablespoons jojoba oil

10 drops lavender (analgesic—numbs pain; regenerates skin cells; reduces sun spots; nurturing, anti-inflammatory, balancing)

3 drops peppermint (cooling, anti-inflammatory, analgesic)

Thoroughly blend all oils together.

Gently apply to all body parts that have been burned and/or exposed to too much sun. Apply as needed for the next 2–3 days.

ESSENTIAL OILS TIP

Keep this blend close at hand when you go to the beach, or just spend a day in the sun. If you follow this protocol you may just be pleasantly surprised that you will have prevented blisters from forming and instead have a healthy glow.

91. CUTS

Ouch! Cuts are a common occurrence. The good news is we can treat them all the same and effectively with our essential oils!

First, clean the area with warm water. Then, add 1 drop each of **lavender** and **tea tree** to the gauze part of an adhesive bandage. Apply directly on top of the cut. Change daily using the same formula and by the third or fourth day, let the air have its turn to help heal.

The blend of lavender and tea tree will work together as an antiseptic, anti-infectious, anti-bacterial, pain numbing, and anti-inflammatory mixture, while emotionally giving you some calmness and nurturing.

92. BRUISING

If you have been injured deeply into the muscle tissue, please first seek appropriate medical attention. Bruises can indicate a more serious injury.

The color of a bruise will change as it heals—red, blue, and purple; then green to yellow. What has happened is blood has found an escape route outside of the vessels and has entered the surrounding tissue.

If you have access to ice, apply it directly to the bruise to prevent further swelling. You can keep the ice 15 minutes on, 15 minutes off for about an hour until you can touch the bruise without excessive pain.

Then prepare this blend of essential oils to make a compress:

2 tablespoons jojoba or grape seed oil
5 drops geranium (cooling, anti-inflammatory; rejuvenates skin cells; promotes blood circulation)
8 drops lavender (analgesic—numbs pain; anti-inflammatory; rejuvenates skin cells)

Thoroughly blend all oils.

Add 8 drops of the blend to 2 cups cold water. Add a cloth to the water and oil mixture and allow it to completely soak in all of the blend. Wring out excess water and apply directly on top of the bruise and leave on until the cloth feels warm. Reapply every 2–3 hours until the bruise begins to decrease in size.

93. SCARRING

The life of a scar begins with an injury. There are scars from burns, falling, surgery . . . the list goes on. The degree of trauma to the body will impact how the body repairs itself. As the body is healing, a tissue of skin forms over the wound as a scar. In time, its size and redness will decrease, but it will probably leave a permanent mark on your skin. Sometimes scars can be painful for a long time.

Some people want to reduce or remove scars and use chemical treatments or even surgery. The therapeutic properties of essential oils not only support the healing process but also assist with tissue repair and cell regeneration. It will take time, but if you patiently apply them every day, you will see a difference.

WHAT SCAR?

2 tablespoons jojoba oil

1 capsule vitamin E (antioxidant; protects and repairs)

3 drops frankincense (cytophylactic—protects existing cells and encourages new cell growth)

3 drops geranium (promotes blood circulation to area of injury, reducing scar tissue)

7 drops lavender (regenerates skin cells; tightens skin; reduces scarring)

Using a sterile sharp pin, puncture a vitamin E capsule and add the contents to the jojoba oil. Then add the remaining oils and thoroughly blend. Apply directly over the scar up to 2 times a day until the scar subsides. Remember, it may take a couple months to see a difference, so be patient and use every day. Keep oils stored in a dark glass container that can be tightly sealed.

94. NAIL FUNGUS

Incorporating essential oils into your life will result in benefits that range from the immediate to the long-term. For example, you may discover your nails are strong, healthy, and growing at a faster rate than before. It's important to take care of the nail bed and cuticle. When a doctor or integrative health practitioner is interested in your current state of health, he or she will look at your nail color (without polish), texture, and any white spots. At times, however, a nail fungus appears on either the hands or feet. When a fungus is active and left unattended, the nail may turn deep yellowish and become very thick. At this point, the nail is very hard to cut and may require the attention of a medical professional.

Let's use our essential oils to make a small blend to take good care of our nails and one to make in case we have nail fungus. We will be working with **lavender, lemon,** and **tea tree**.

NOURISHED NAILS

1 tablespoon grape seed oil

1 tablespoon jojoba oil

8 drops lavender (antiseptic, antibacterial; rejuvenates new cell growth)

3 drops lemon (bactericide, disinfectant, antiseptic; soothing to dry skin)

Thoroughly blend all oils.

Use on and around your nails and cuticles. Only apply about 1 drop of blend for each nail. Use on both hands and feet. Store in a dark glass container with a tight fitting lid.

FAREWELL FUNGUS

1 tablespoon grape seed oil

1 tablespoon jojoba oil

7 drops lavender (antiseptic, antibacterial; rejuvenates new cell growth)

7 drops tea tree (anti-infectious, antifungal, antibacterial)

Thoroughly blend all oils.

Apply 1–2 drops of the blend on top of and under the nail. Use a dropper as needed. You can apply this in the morning and evening.

ESSENTIAL OILS TIP

Many have found success using tea tree oil "neat" (without dilution) directly on the nail(s) infected. Drop the oil directly on the fungus and around the nail bed and cuticle. Do this twice a day.

95. DANDRUFF

That little black dress is stunning! You're all set to have a great time until these little white dots on the shoulders of your dress catch your eye. Excusing yourself, you go into the bathroom and brush off the dead skin cells that you thought you had under control. Why can't anybody come up with a hair product to eliminate dandruff?

Let's take control of our hair care using essential oils. Before shampooing your hair, support the scalp with some conditioning:

DANDRUFF CONDITIONING TREATMENT

2 tablespoons jojoba oil

2 drops clary sage

4 drops lavender

4 drops tea tree

1 drop ylang ylang

Blend all oils together.

Wet your hair, apply the treatment, and leave on for 20–30 minutes. Be sure to reach your scalp with this blend, not just your hair. Then, wash your hair as normal.

ESSENTIAL OILS TIP

Make your own dandruff shampoo by adding 10 drops of lavender, 10 drops of tea tree, and 2 drops of ylang ylang to 8 ounces of a high-quality, organic shampoo.

96. DRY HAIR

Dry hair is dull, lifeless, and challenging to style. It is brittle and easily breaks, tangles, and splits. The reasons for dry hair vary from our health and environment to our hair-styling tools and products. If you have been challenged for some time with dry hair, you may want to get a medical checkup to see how your hormones are balancing. If all is well, then you can put some essential oils to work.

Three excellent oils from this book are **geranium, lavender,** and **rosemary**.

HOT OIL HAIR TREATMENT

2 tablespoons jojoba oil

1 drop geranium

1 drop lavender

1 drop rosemary

Heat water to almost the boiling point in a small pan on a stove. When warm, add a small heat resistant bowl inside pan.

Add jojoba oil inside the smaller bowl to warm the oil. Add the drops of geranium, lavender, and rosemary. Thoroughly blend all oils.

Separate hair into 4 sections, and working with one section at a time, saturate with the oil mixture using a fine-toothed comb.

When all hair is saturated with oil, place a plastic shower cap on your head and wrap with a warm towel. (You can always tumble a towel in the dryer for a couple minutes to warm.) Leave on your hair for 30 minutes.

Shampoo your hair a minimum of 2 times to completely remove all the oil. If you want to add a small amount of baking soda to your shampoo, this will help eliminate the excess oil and leave your hair really clean. You can use the Hot Oil Hair Treatment once a week.

ESSENTIAL OILS TIP

The 30 minutes your hot oil treatment is working would be a great time to do a facial steam as outlined in Section 79 of this book. You and your hair will be radiant!

If you have epilepsy, are prone to seizures, are pregnant, and/or breastfeeding, do not use rosemary.

97. FRAGILE HAIR

The difference between dry and fragile hair is that fragile hair is the end result of abusing hair products and styling tools. When an overload of chemicals and heat are used on the hair consistently, it becomes fragile and breaks at the slightest touch. The first thing, then, is to eliminate harsh chemicals. You can replace them with pure essential oils to nurture the remaining cells back to health and allow new growth to prosper. We will work with lavender and clary sage along with jojoba oil.

FRAGILE HAIR REPAIR HOT OIL TREATMENT

2 tablespoons jojoba oil

1 drop clary sage

1 drop lavender

Heat water to almost the boiling point in a small pan on a stove. When warm, add a small heat resistant bowl inside pan.

Add jojoba oil inside the smaller bowl to warm the oil. Add the drops of clary sage and lavender. Thoroughly blend all oils.

Separate hair into 4 sections, and working with one section at a time, saturate the hair with the oil mixture using a fine-toothed comb.

When all the hair is saturated with oil, place a plastic shower cap on your head and wrap with a warm towel. (You can always tumble a towel in the dryer for a couple minutes to warm.). Leave on hair for 30 minutes.

Shampoo your hair a minimum of 2 times to completely remove all the oil. If you want to add a small amount of baking soda to your shampoo, this will help eliminate the excess oil and leave your hair really clean. Follow with conditioner. You can do the Fragile Hair Repair Hot Oil Treatment weekly.

If you can locate an organic, unscented gentle shampoo and conditioner, for every 4 ounces, add two drops each of lavender and clary sage.

ESSENTIAL OILS TIP

After you towel dry your hair, be very careful handling the hair. Wet hair can be damaged or broken very easily. The best thing to do first is run your fingers gently through your hair, and follow with a large-tooth comb or a brush specifically designed to smooth out wet hair.

98. STOPPING HAIR LOSS

It is very normal to lose up to 100 hairs per day. However, if there is a history of family hair loss, or you are under a lot of stress, your diet is poor, you are aging, or perhaps you have thyroid challenges, then hair loss will exceed the normal rate and may cause concern along with low self-esteem. If you feel you have a hormonal or medical challenge, then first address that with the proper professional care.

Try not to wash your hair daily as this may aggravate the loss. If possible, wash your hair up to three times a week—no more. We will work with the essential oils of **lavender** and **rosemary** for this section, along with some jojoba oil for the blends.

Purchase a shampoo and conditioner that is vegetable based and unscented. Then you can add the oils as follows:

For every 8 ounces of shampoo and conditioner add the following:

1 teaspoon jojoba oil (shampoo only)
12 drops lavender
10 drops rosemary

Thoroughly blend all ingredients and use as normal. You can always adjust the oils to your liking. Do not use more than 24 drops per one cup of shampoo or conditioner.

If you have epilepsy, are prone to seizures, are pregnant, and/or breastfeeding, do not use rosemary.

99. STIMULATING HAIR GROWTH

If you have hair follicles, there's every reason to positively work toward regrowth. There is always the possibility of losing your hair even after it has grown out, but consider giving essential oils a try. They cannot harm the hair follicles and will enhance them if possible.

We will be blending a scalp massage to be used every day. Jojoba oil will be our base for **clary sage, lavender, lemon,** and **rosemary** essential oils.

HAIR WE GO!

2 tablespoons jojoba oil (moisturizes hair, adds nutrients, stimulates scalp)

3 drops clary sage (promotes hair growth, stimulates scalp)

6 drops lavender (deep conditions hair, promotes hair growth)

2 drops lemon (stimulates underactive sebaceous glands)

3 drops rosemary (stimulates roots, increases circulation, improves hair growth)

Thoroughly blend all oils.

Place the blended oils in the palms of your hands and rub together. Use both hands and massage the oils onto the *scalp* of head, not the hair. Your hair will get some oils, but it is your scalp that needs attention. Do not rub the scalp, but massage it to stimulate the blood circulation in the vessels. This is extremely important for hair growth stimulation. Massage your scalp for a couple of minutes and then put on a plastic shower cap and cover with a towel for 30–45 minutes. Shampoo and rinse hair as normal.

ESSENTIAL OILS TIP

You can add the following to 8 ounces of your shampoo:

One teaspoon jojoba oil, 6 drops clary sage, 14 drops lavender, 6 drops lemon, and 6 drops rosemary. Omit rosemary if you are pregnant and/or breastfeeding, have epilepsy, or are prone to seizures.

100. SHAMPOO AND CONDITIONER

If you have ever wanted to make your own shampoo and conditioner you have come to the right place! These recipes are very basic and adaptable per your unique hair needs.

SHAMPOO

½ cup liquid castile soap

½ cup distilled water

1 tablespoon jojoba oil

20 drops of essential oils of your choice (listed)

Thoroughly blend all ingredients and store them in either a flip- or squirt-top plastic bottle (PET). This will make 8 ounces. If you want larger sizes, just combine equal amounts of castile soap and water and increase the jojoba and essential oils accordingly. This shampoo is not "lathery" but will do an excellent job. You will actually use less. Follow with conditioner:

CONDITIONER

1 cup water

1 tablespoon apple cider vinegar

20 drops essential oils of your choice (listed)

Thoroughly blend all ingredients and store in an 8-ounce plastic (PET) bottle with a flip or squirt top. Use after each shampoo.

The following is a list of essential oils from this book for hair care. Choose the ones that suit your particular needs.

■ All Hair Types: Clary sage, lavender

■ Dandruff: Clary sage, eucalyptus, lavender, lemon, rosemary, tea tree, ylang ylang

■ Oily: Clary sage, lavender, lemon, rosemary, tea tree, ylang ylang

■ Dry: Clary sage, lavender, lemon, peppermint, tea tree

■ Hair Growth: Clary sage, lavender, peppermint, rosemary, ylang ylang

Caution: Do not use essential oils directly on the hair without diluting first in either water, shampoo and or carrier oil.

ESSENTIAL OILS TIP

If you don't want to make your own shampoo or conditioner, purchase unscented, natural ones at your local health food store or order online. Then, add the essential oils of your choice. For every 8 ounces add a combined total of 20 drops of essential oils.

If you have epilepsy, are prone to seizures, are pregnant, and/or breastfeeding, do not use rosemary.

INDEX

ABOUT THE AUTHOR

Kymberly Keniston-Pond is the owner of Kymberly's LLC. That business reflects her accomplishments as an artist; Certified Integrative Reflexologist; Certified Clinical Master Aromatherapist; developer of an organic skin care line, Earthen Beauty; and a Continued Education Provider for reflexology and aromatherapy. Though she works with all people, her passion is working with women and persons with disabilities. She holds four reflexology certifications, three reflexology diplomas from Sorensen Institute in Spain, and three aromatherapy certifications, inclusive of her Clinical Master Aromatherapy. In addition, she holds a TCGI Grant Writing Certification and a Certification for Supporting Adults with ASDs.

She has been a presenter for the Virginia Community Colleges Association's annual concurrent sessions in 2009 and 2010, as well as a presenter in 2010 for Therapeutic Recreation for her work using essential oils with people with disabilities. She has appeared on the *Virginia This Morning* television program, been published in *Natural Awakenings* magazine, and was featured in Richmond's *Belle* magazine. Contact her at *wildflowersart@yahoo.com*.